Clinical Trials in Stargardt Disease Treatment

Jeffrey N. Weiss

Clinical Trials in Stargardt Disease Treatment

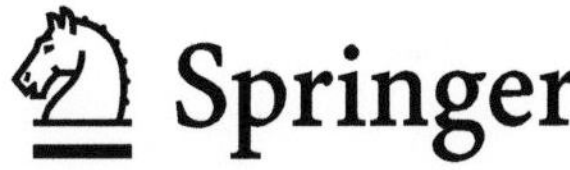 Springer

Jeffrey N. Weiss
Parkland, FL, USA

ISBN 978-3-031-58809-9   ISBN 978-3-031-58807-5   (eBook)
https://doi.org/10.1007/978-3-031-58807-5

This Springer imprint is published by the registered company Springer Nature Switzerland AG
The registered company address is: Gewerbestrasse 11, 6330 Cham, Switzerland

If disposing of this product, please recycle the paper.

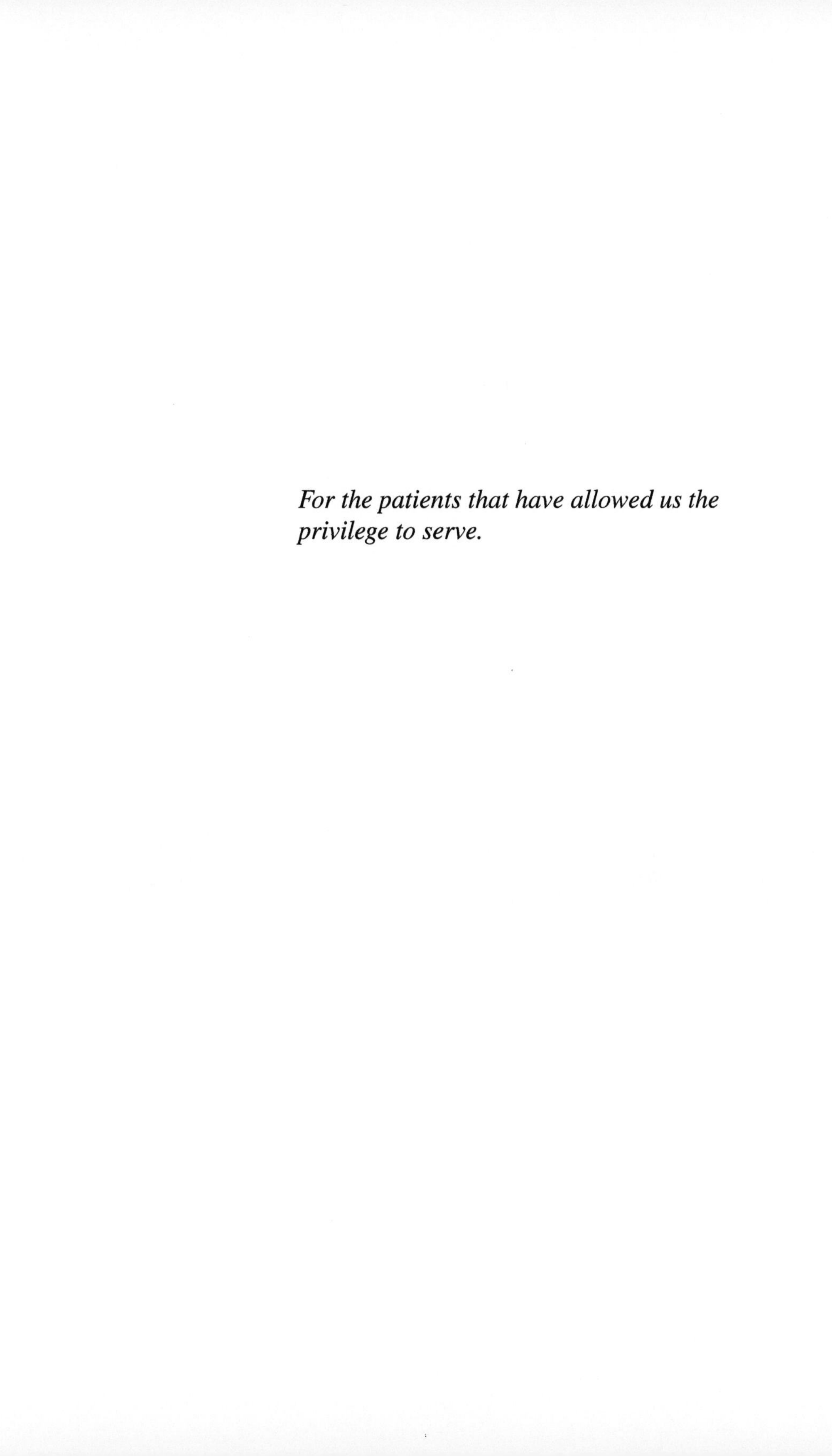

For the patients that have allowed us the privilege to serve.

Preface

This book is a compendium of the worldwide ocular stem cell, gene therapy, pharmaceutical, and other miscellaneous studies treating Stargardt disease registered with Clinicaltrials.gov. Clinicaltrials.gov is the largest website listing of registered clinical research studies in the world.

The information presented is accurate as of November 2023. I have divided the studies into multiple categories: Completed, Active/Recruiting, Active/Not-Recruiting, Not Yet Recruiting, and Enrolling by Invitation. Regarding study location, United States locations are listed first, followed by other countries in alphabetical order. As studies have many testing sites, frequently in many countries, the sponsor location is used.

I corrected the mischaracterization of studies, only included those that truly belonged within each category, removed extraneous information, and corrected spelling and grammar, in order to produce a consistent and easy-to-read format. The Study and the Clinical Trial number are provided to make it easier for the reader to obtain further information.

I hope that by providing this reference, the field of Stargardt disease treatment will be advanced.

Parkland, FL, USA   Jeffrey N. Weiss

Contents

Chapter 1
Introduction to Stargardt Disease

Karl Stargardt (1875–1927) was a German ophthalmologist and the Chairman of the Department of Ophthalmology at the University of Marburg. In 1909, he described 7 patients with a recessively inherited macular dystrophy and progressive and severe visual loss beginning in the Tables first two decades of life. The eponymous Stargardt disease (STGD) is the most common form of inherited juvenile macular degeneration with a prevalence of 1 to 8000–10,000. There is an association with several different genes:

STGD1: the most common type (95% of cases) is autosomal recessive and caused by mutations in the ABCA4 gene, although it can also be associated with a mutation in CNGB3. Defective ABCA4 affects the ATP-binding cassette transporter protein causing the formation of toxic vitamin A biretinoids. Damaged retinal cells will form lipofuscin in the retinal pigment epithelium, the characteristic finding in this condition. There are over 1000 mutations of ABCA4 known to cause STGD1 and related retinal diseases.

STGD2 was discontinued when it was discovered to be caused by the same gene as STGD3.

STGD3: This is a rare dominant type of Stargardt disease caused by a mutation in the ELOVL4 gene.

STGD4: This type is associated with mutations in PROM1.

Efforts to address the lack of therapy for Stargardt disease have included oral therapy, intravitreal injections, stem cells, and gene therapy.

ALK-001 is a synthetic vitamin A once-a-day pill that prevents the formation of toxic vitamin A dimers in the eye. This form of vitamin A is not readily converted to lipofuscin, slowing its deposition and potentially slowing vision loss. ALK-001 and other vitamin A variants are being explored. However, oral intake of excessive vitamin A has been shown to increase lipofuscin deposition in animal models, possibly worsening the loss of vision in Stargardt disease.

J. N. Weiss, *Clinical Trials in Stargardt Disease Treatment*, https://doi.org/10.1007/978-3-031-58807-5_1

There are several surgical treatments reported:

1. Ocata therapeutics (previously Advanced Cell Technology) has completed a multicenter trial using retinal pigment epithelial cells derived from human embryonic stem cells. No ocular safety issues were encountered, though side effects from patient immunosuppression were observed. The company was subsequently acquired by Astellas Pharma and follow-up studies are continuing.
2. The Stem Cell Ophthalmology Treatment Study (SCOTS and SCOTS2) reported treating 34 eyes with Stargardt disease using autologous bone marrow-derived stem cells. With a one-year follow-up period, 21 (61.8%) improved, 8 (23.5%) remained stable, and 5 (14.7%) showed continued progression of their disease. The results were statistically significant with $p = 0.0004$. The average central vision improvement following treatment was 17.96% (95%CI, 16.39–19.53%) and ranged up to 80.5%. Of 17 patients treated, 13 (76.5%) showed visual acuity improvement in one or both eyes, 3 patients (17.6%) showed no net loss, and 1 worsened as a consequence of disease progression; 94.1% of patients had improved vision or remained stable. There were no adverse events.

The explanation for using stem cells to treat patients with visual acuity loss of a genetic etiology is that the stem cells may benefit damaged but repairable cells via neuroprotection mechanisms, reduce ongoing immunogenic damage, transfer cytoplasmic structures including mitochondria and lysosomes to damaged cells, and produce neuronal transformation which can fuse with Müller cells to then transdifferentiate into specialized neurons including ganglion and amacrine neurons.

The ABCA4 transporter is located primarily in the retina and is one of multiple ABCA proteins associated with lipid transport across cell membranes. It is responsible for transporting N-retinylidene-PE from the lumen to the cytoplasmic side of the disc membrane, allowing conversion of all-trans retinal to all-trans retinol, which is then transported into the RPE (Retinal Pigment Epithelial) cells. There it converts to 11-cis retinal, which is transported back into the outer segment of the photoreceptor to combine with opsin and regenerate rhodopsin or cone opsin completing the visual cycle.

With an abnormal ABCA4 transporter, removal of the N-retinylidene-PE is impaired which allows it to react with all-trans retinal to form a derivative called A2PE. Because outer segments of the photoreceptors are constantly renewed, RPE cells ingest the A2PE in phagosomes which fuse with lysosomes to degrade. However, A2PE can only be hydrolyzed to N-retinylidene-N-retinyl-ethanolamine (A2E) and cannot be further broken down. A2E accumulates progressively in the RPE cells as a component of lipofuscin. Lipofuscin is a complex combination of oxidized macromolecules which can accumulate in different tissues. With blue light exposure, lipofuscin in the RPE can form epoxides which can cause RPE apoptosis. Ultimately, RPE cell death causes photoreceptor cell death and decreased vision.

The purpose of gene replacement therapy is to attempt to decrease or stop additional retinal tissue loss by targeting photoreceptors. Though the most experience had been obtained with Adeno-associated virus vectors, the ABCA4 gene is larger than the capacity of the current AAV vector, which makes the lentivirus the vector of choice. A lentivirus vector is being tested.

The multicenter Natural History of the Progression of Atrophy Secondary to Stargardt Disease studies describe the natural history of disease progression. The study determined that the rate of progression was mainly determined by the initial lesion size.

Further Reading

Adler L IV, Boyer NP, Chen C, Ablonczy Z, Crouch RK, Koutalos Y. The 11-cis retinal origins of lipofuscin in the retina. Prog Mol Biol Transl Sci. 2015;134:e1–12. https://doi.org/10.1016/bs.pmbts.2015.07.022. ISBN 9780128010594. PMID 26310175.

Audo I, Weleber R, Stout T, Lauer AK, Pennesi ME, Mohand-Said S, Barale P-O, Buggage R, Wilson DJ, Sahel JA. Early findings in a phase I/IIa clinical program for Stargardt disease. Investig Ophthalmol Vis Sci. 2015;56:3819.

Campa C, Gallenga CE, Bolletta E, Perri P. The role of gene therapy in the treatment of retinal diseases: A review. Curr Gene Ther. 2017;17:194–213.

Cideciyan AV, Swider M, Aleman TS, Tsybovsky Y, Schwartz SB, Windsor EA, et al. ABCA4 disease progression and a proposed strategy for gene therapy. Hum Mol Genet. 2009;18(5):931–41. https://doi.org/10.1093/hmg/ddn421. PMC 2640207. PMID 19074458.

Dalkara D, Goureau O, Marazova K, Sahel JA. Let there be light: gene and cell therapy for blindness. Hum Gene Ther. 2016;27:134–47.

Deutman A, Hoyng C, van Lith-Verhoeven J. Macular dystrophies. In: Retina. 4th ed. Elsevier Mosby; 2006. p. 1171–4.

Fakin A, Robson AG, Fujinami K, Moore AT, Michaelides M, Pei-Wen Chiang J, et al. Phenotype and progression of retinal degeneration associated with nullizigosity of ABCA4. Invest Ophthalmol Vis Sci. 2016;57(11):4668–78. https://doi.org/10.1167/iovs.16-19829. PMID 27583828. S2CID 23322124.

Fujinami K, Lois N, Davidson AE, Mackay DS, Hogg CR, Stone EM, Tsunoda K, Tsubota K, Bunce C, Robson AG, et al. A longitudinal study of Stargardt disease: clinical and electrophysiologic assessment, progression, and genotype correlations. Am J Ophthalmol. 2013;155:1075–88.

Fujinami K, Zernat J, Chana RK, Wright GA, Tsunoda K, Ozawa Y, Tsubota K, Robson AG, Holder GE, Allikmets R, et al. Clinical and molecular characteristics of childhood-onset Stargardt disease. Ophthalmology. 2015;122:326–34.

Ibanez MB IV, de Guimaraes TA, Capasso J, Bello N, Levin AV. Stargardt misdiagnosis: How ocular genetics helps. Am J Med Genet A. 2021;185(3):814–9. https://doi.org/10.1002/ajmg.a.62045. ISSN 1552-4825. PMID 33369172. S2CID 229691125.

Jimenez-Rolando B, Noval S, Rosa-Peres I, Diaz EM, Del Pozo A, Ibañez C, Silla JC, Montaño VEF, Martin-Arenas R, Vallespin E. Next generation sequencing in the diagnosis of Stargardt's disease. Arch Soc Esp Oftalmol. 2018;93:119–25.

Kong X, West SK, Strauss RW, Munoz B, Cideciyan AV, Michaelides M, Ho A, Ahmed M, Schönbach EM, Cheetham JK, et al. Progression of visual acuity and fundus autofluorescence in recent-onset Stargardt disease: ProgStar study report #4. Ophthalmol Retin. 2017;1:514–23.

Kubota R, Birch DG, Gregory JK, Koester JM. Randomised study evaluating the pharmacodynamics of emixustat hydrochloride in subjects with macular atrophy secondary to Stargardt disease. Br J Ophthalmol. 2020;106(3):403–8. https://doi.org/10.1136/bjophthalmol-2020-317712. ISSN 0007-1161. PMC 8867285. PMID 33214244.

Molday RS, Zhong M, Quazi F. The role of the photoreceptor ABC transporter ABCA4 in lipid transport and Stargardt macular degeneration. Biochim Biophys Acta. 2009;1791:573–83.

Pesaresi M, Bonilla-Pons SA, Simonte G, Sanges D, Di Vicino U, Cosma MP. Endogenous mobilization of bone-marrow cells into the murine retina induces fusion-mediated reprogramming of Muller glia cells. EBioMedicine. 2018;30:38–51.

Pfau M, Holz FG, Müller PL. Retinal light sensitivity as outcome measure in recessive Stargardt disease. Br J Ophthalmol. 2021;105(2):258–64. https://doi.org/10.1136/bjophthalmol-2020-316201. PMID 32345606. S2CID 216645815.

Pfau M, Cukras CA, Huryn LA, Zein WM, Ullah E, Boyle MP, et al. Photoreceptor degeneration in ABCA4-associated retinopathy and its genetic correlates. JCI Insight. 2022;7(2) https://doi.org/10.1172/jci.insight.155373. PMC 8855828. PMID 35076026.

Schwartz SD, Regillo CD, Lam BL, Eliott D, Rosenfeld PJ, Gregori NZ, Hubschman J-P, Davis JL, Heilwell G, Spirn M, et al. Human embryonic stem cell-derived retinal pigment epithelium in patients with age-related macular degenerations and Stargardt's macular dystrophy:follow-up of two open-label phase 1/2 studies. Lancet. 2015;385:509–16.

Stargardt KB. Über familiäre, progressive Degeneration in der Makulagegend des Auges. Albrecht von Graefes Archiv für Ophthalmologie (in German). 1909;71(3):534–50. https://doi.org/10.1007/BF01961301. S2CID 12557316.

Strauss RW, Munoz B, Ho A, Jha A, Michaelides M, Cideciyan AV, Audo I, Birch DG, Hariri AH, Nittala MG, et al. Progression of Stargardt disease as determined by fundus autofluorescence in the retrospective progression of Stargardt disease study (ProgStar report no. 9). JAMA Ophthalmol. 2017;135:1232–41.

Tanna P, Strauss RW, Gujinami K, Michaelides M. Stargardt disease: clinical features, molecular genetics, animal models and therapeutic options. Br J Ophthalmol. 2017;101:25–30.

Trapani I. Dual AAV vectors for Stargardt disease. Methods Mol Biol. 2018;1715:153–75.

Travis GH, Golczak M, Moise AR, Palczewski K. Diseases caused by defects in the visual cycle: Retinoids as potential therapeutic agents. Annu Rev Pharmacol Toxicol. 2007;47:469–512.

Waugh N, Loveman E, Colquitt J, Royle P. Treatments for dry age-related macular degeneration and Stargardt disease: a systematic review. Health Technol Assess. 2018;22:1–168.

Weiss JN, Levy S. Stem cell ophthalmology treatment study (SCOTS): Bone marrow-derived stem cells in the treatment of stargardt disease. Medicines (Basel, Switzerland). 2021;8(2):10. https://doi.org/10.3390/medicines8020010. ISSN 2305-6320. PMC 7913552. PMID 33546345.

Chapter 2
Tables

See Tables 2.1, 2.2, 2.3, and 2.4

Table 2.1 Active studies

	UNITED STATES	AUSTRALIA	SPAIN	SWITZERLAND
TOTAL NUMBER OF STUDIES	15	1	1	1
NON-PROPRIETARY	6		1	1
PROPRIETARY	8	1		
SUPPORT				
CORPORATE	8	1		
UNIVERSITY/HOSPITAL/MD			1	1
NEI	6			
NONPROFIT	1			
NO SUPPORT	1			
Phase Not Applicable	7		1	1
Phase 1				
Phase 1/2	3	1		
Phase 2	4			
Phase 2/3				
Phase 3	1			

© The Author(s), under exclusive license to Springer Nature
Switzerland AG 2024
J. N. Weiss, *Clinical Trials in Stargardt Disease Treatment*,
https://doi.org/10.1007/978-3-031-58807-5_2

Table 2.2 Completed studies

	UNITED STATES	BRAZIL	CHINA	COLUMBIA	EUROPE	UNITED KINGDOM	NO LOCATION
TOTALNUMBER OF STUDIES	11	1	1	1	2	2	1
NONPROPRIETARY	5		1	1	2		
PROPRIETARY	6	1				2	1
SUPPORT							
CORPORATE	5	1				2	1
UNIVERSITY/HOSPITAL/MD	4		1	1	2		
NEI	1						
NONPROFIT	1						
NO SUPPORT							
Phase Not Applicable	4		1	1			
Phase 1	3						1
Phase 1/2	2	1				2	
Phase 2	3						
Phase 2/3							
Phase 3	1						

Table 2.3 Terminated/unknown studies

	UNITED STATES	CHINA	EUROPE	KOREA	UNITED KINGDOM
TOTAL NUMBER OF STUDIES	3	1	2	1	1
NON-PROPRIETARY	2	1	2		1
PROPRIETARY	1			1	
SUPPORT					
CORPORATE	1			1	
UNIVERSITY/HOSPITAL/MD	2	1	2		1
NEI					
NONPROFIT					
NO SUPPORT					
Phase Not Applicable	2		1		1
Phase 1			1	1	
Phase 1/2	1	1			
Phase 2					
Phase 2/3					
Phase 3					

Table 2.4 All studies (Except terminated and unknown)

	UNITED STATES	AUSTRALIA	CHINA	EUROPE	NO LOCATION	SOUTH AMERICA	SPAIN	SWITZERLAND
NUMBER OF STUDIES	27	1	1	4	1	2	1	1
DRUGS	15	1		1	1			
ELECTRICAL	1							
SURGERY	2			1		1		
OBSERVATION/FU	3			1				
TESTING	3			1				
NATURAL HISTORY	3						1	1
TRAINING			1					
ACUPUNCTURE						1		

Chapter 3
Recruiting Studies

Recruiting

United States

Study to Assess the Safety and Efficacy of OCU410ST for Stargardt Disease (GARDian)

ClinicalTrials.gov ID NCT05956626

Sponsor Ocugen
Information provided by Ocugen (Responsible Party)
Last Update Posted 2023-10-25

Study Overview

Brief Summary
This is a Phase 1/2 Study to Assess the Safety and Efficacy of OCU410ST for Stargardt Disease.

This is a multicenter study, which will be conducted in two phases and will enroll up to a total of 42 subjects.

Detailed Description
Name of Investigational Product: OCU410ST Name of Active Ingredient: Adeno-associated viral vector 5 human RORA (AAV5-hRORA)

Title of Study
A Phase 1/2 Study to Assess the Safety and Efficacy of OCU410ST for Stargardt Disease.

Study Center(s)
Approximately five clinical study centers in the US.

J. N. Weiss, *Clinical Trials in Stargardt Disease Treatment*,
https://doi.org/10.1007/978-3-031-58807-5_3

Background

Stargardt disease is an eye disease that causes vision loss in children and young adults. It is an inherited disease caused by faulty genes that cause build up of fat deposits in the eye. Currently, there is no approved treatment available for Stargardt disease.

OCU410ST Product Information

OCU410ST is an Adeno-Associated Virus serotype 5 containing human RORA for the treatment of Stargardt disease. Dysregulation in lipid metabolism, oxidative stress, and anti-inflammatory mechanisms are critical for pathogenesis and progression of Stargardt disease. The role of hRORA in regulating these gene pathways strongly suggests that OCU410ST could restore homeostasis in the eye and thereby serve as a therapeutic candidate for Stargardt disease.

This study will be conducted in two phases enrolling up to 42 subjects.

Phase 1 is a multicenter, open-label, dose-ranging/dose escalation study with a 3+3 design enrolling up to 18 subjects

Phase 2 is a randomized, dose-expansion cohort in which 24 subjects will be randomized in a 1:1:1 ratio into either one of two treatment groups (adults and pediatric subjects) or to an untreated (adults and pediatric subjects) control group.

Official Title

A Phase 1/2 Study to Assess the Safety and Efficacy of OCU410ST for STARGARDT DISEASE

Conditions

Stargardt Disease

Intervention/Treatment

- Genetic: OCU410ST

Other Study ID Numbers

- OCU410ST-101

Study Start (Actual)

2023-08-25

Primary Completion (Estimated)

2025-10-28

Study Completion (Estimated)

2025-10-28

Enrollment (Estimated)

42

Study Type

Interventional

Phase

Phase 1 and Phase 2

Study Contact
Name: Umair Qazi, MD, MPH
Phone Number: +1 (202)-817-0787
Email: umair.qazi@ocugen.com
Study Contact Backup
Name: Mahvish Tafseer, MD, ACRP-CP
Phone Number: +1 (215) 934-8891
Email: mahvish.tafseer@ocugen.com

United States
Texas Locations

Bellaire, Texas, United States, 77401
Recruiting
Retina Consultants of Texas

Contact
Rebbecca Tiang
800-833-5921 rebbecca.taing@retinaconsultantstexas.com
Principal Investigator:
Charles Wykoff, MD, PhD

Dallas, Texas, United States, 75231
Recruiting
Retina Foundation of the Southwest

Contact
Kimberly Cummings, CCRC
214-363-3911 ext 128 evasquez@retinafoundation.org
Principal Investigator:
Karl Csaky, MD, PhD

Eligibility Criteria
Description

Inclusion Criteria
- Are aged 18–65.
- Have clinical evidence of a macular lesion phenotypically consistent with Stargardt Disease
- The study eye should have at least one well-demarcated area of atrophy with a minimum diameter of 300 microns and total lesion size <= 18 mmE2 and a BCVA of 50 ETDRS letters or better
- Have confirmed presence of two pathogenic mutations in the ABCA4 gene
- Have detectable outer nuclear layer (ONL) in the macular region tomography (SD-OCT).
- Have BCVA of 50 letters or less (using ETDRS chart)

Key Inclusion Criteria for Pediatric Subjects
- Are aged 6–17.
- Have clinical diagnosis of Stargardt Disease
- The designated primary study eye must have at least one well-demarcated area of atrophy with a minimum diameter of 300 microns and a total lesion area <= 18 mmE2 and a BCVA of 35 ETDRS letters or better.
- Have two (2) pathogenic mutations confirmed present, in the ABCA4 gene.

Key Exclusion Criteria for Adult Subjects
- Have previous treatment with a gene therapy or cell therapy product.
- Have any concurrent retroviral therapy that would inactivate the investigational product.
- Have any contradictions for subretinal injection and the use of anesthesia.
- Have genes that mimic Stargardt Disease, like ELOVL4 or PROM1.

Exclusion Criteria for Pediatric Subjects
- Have previous treatment with a gene therapy or cell therapy product.
- Have any concurrent retroviral therapy that would inactivate the investigational product.
- Have any intraocular surgery (including lens replacement surgery) within 6 months (prior to Screening) and any ophthalmic condition that may require surgery during the study period.
- Have genes that mimic Stargardt Disease, like ELOVL4 or PROM1.

Ages Eligible for Study
6–65 Years (Child, Adult, Older Adult)

Sexes Eligible for Study
All

Accepts Healthy Volunteers
No

Design Details
Primary Purpose: Treatment
Allocation: Randomized
Interventional Model: Sequential Assignment

Interventional Model Description
The study will be conducted in two phases.

Phase 1 is a multicenter, open-label, dose-ranging/dose escalation study. A 3+3 study design will be used for the sequential dose-escalation cohorts in which subjects will receive a single subretinal injection of OCU410ST.

Phase 2 is a dose-expansion phase of the study, where the subjects will be randomized in a 1:1:1 ratio to either one of two treatment groups (adult and pediatric subjects) or to an untreated (adult and pediatric subjects) control group.

Masking: Single (Outcomes Assessor)
Masking Description:
The following team members will be masked:
Bio-Statistician, Data Programmer, Imaging Reading Center Team, Head of Clinical Development, and Medical Affairs.

Arms and interventions

Participant group/arm	Intervention/treatment
Experimental: Experimental: Phase1 Dose Escalation- Low Dose (3.75 × 10E10 vg/mL): Low Dose (3.75 × 10E10 vg/mL): Subjects will receive a subretinal injection of 200 µL of OCU410ST in the low dose concentration.	Genetic: OCU410ST • Subretinal Administration of OCU410ST
Experimental: Experimental: Phase1 Dose Escalation- Medium Dose (7.5 × 10E10 vg/mL): Medium Dose (7.5 × 10E10 vg/mL): Subjects will receive a subretinal injection of OCU410ST in the Medium dose concentration.	Genetic: OCU410ST • Subretinal Administration of OCU410ST
Experimental: Experimental: Phase1 Dose Escalation- High Dose (2.25 × 10E11 vg/mL): High Dose (2.25 × 10E11 vg/mL): Subjects will receive a subretinal injection of OCU410ST in the high-dose concentration.	Genetic: OCU410ST • Subretinal Administration of OCU410ST
Experimental: Experimental: Phase 2 Dose Expansion: Dose 1 from Phase 1-Randomized Adult Arm Subjects will receive a subretinal injection of OCU410ST with Maximum tolerated dose (MTD) from Phase 1.	Genetic: OCU410ST • Subretinal Administration of OCU410ST
Experimental: Experimental: Phase 2 Dose Expansion: Dose 1 from Phase 1-Randomized Pediatric Arm Subjects will receive a subretinal injection of OCU410ST with Maximum tolerated dose (MTD) from Phase 1.	Genetic: OCU410ST • Subretinal Administration of OCU410ST
Experimental: Experimental: Phase 2 Dose Expansion: Dose 2 from Phase 1-Randomized Adult Arm Subjects will receive a subretinal injection of OCU410ST with Lower Dose than Maximum tolerated dose (MTD) from Phase 1	Genetic: OCU410ST • Subretinal Administration of OCU410ST
Experimental: Experimental: Phase 2 Dose Expansion: Dose 2 from Phase 1-Randomized Pediatric Arm Subjects will receive a subretinal injection of OCU410ST with Lower Dose than Maximum tolerated dose (MTD) from Phase 1	Genetic: OCU410ST • Subretinal Administration of OCU410ST
No Intervention: No Intervention- Randomized Control Adult Arm No Intervention Control Arm: Subject will not receive any active study intervention	
No Intervention: No Intervention- Randomized Control Pediatric Arm No Intervention Control Arm: Subject will not receive any active study intervention	

Primary outcome measures

Outcome measure	Measure description	Time frame
Safety (Participants With Ocular and Non-ocular AEs (Adverse Events) and SAEs (Serious Adverse Events))	The primary endpoint is safety, determined by the number of ocular and non-ocular Study Drug-related adverse events (SDAE), treatment-emergent adverse events (TEAEs), and serious adverse events (SAEs).	12 months (Screening to 12 months post-OCU410ST administration)
Ophthalmic Safety: Change From Baseline in BCVA (Best-Corrected Visual Acuity)	Visual function of the study eye was assessed using the Early Treatment Diabetic Retinopathy Study (ETDRS) Best-Corrected Visual Acuity (BCVA) letter score. A higher score represents better vision.	12 months (Screening to 12 months post-OCU410ST administration)
Ophthalmic Safety: Ophthalmoscope Measurements	We will use Slit-lamp Biomicroscopy to visualize the anatomy of ocular structures before and after subretinal injections and follow-up visits.	12 months (Screening to 12 months post OCU410ST administration)
Ophthalmic Safety: Change in the Intraocular Pressure (mmHg)	Measured by applanation or rebound tonometry with confirmation with Goldmann tonometer if IOP is outside normal range (8–21mmHg).	12 months (Screening to 12 months post-OCU410ST administration)
Change Using Qualitative and quantitative assessments of autofluorescence pattern (FAF)	Changes in the intensity of FAF will be evaluated from the baseline measurements, to assess the loss of retinal layers.	12 months (Screening to 12 months post-OCU410ST administration)
Ophthalmic Safety: Changes in Full Field ERG	The International Society for Clinical Electrophysiology of Vision (ISCEV) guidelines will be followed for conducting ff-ERG (Full-field Electroretinography)	12 months (Screening to 12 months post-OCU410ST administration)

Secondary outcome measures

Outcome measure	Measure description	Time frame
Humoral and cellular immune response	Blood samples will be collected for the assessment. The secondary safety endpoints include change from baseline in Humoral and cellular immune response in response to OCU410ST administration	12 months (Screening to 12 months post-OCU410ST administration)
Shedding of Viral Vector	Blood samples will be collected for the assessment to determine AAV vector shedding in systemic circulation after OCU410ST administration	12 months (Screening to 12 months post-OCU410ST administration)

Outcome measure	Measure description	Time frame
Change in laboratory parameters for Hematology	Blood samples will be collected to determine any significant change in hematology parameters including hematocrit, hemoglobin, red and white blood cell count, and any other parameters deemed necessary by study investigator from baseline after OCU410ST administration.	12 months (Screening to 12 months post-OCU410ST administration)
Change in laboratory parameters for Serum Chemistry	Blood samples will be collected to determine any significant change in serum chemistry parameters including electrolytes, renal functions, liver functions, comprehensive metabolic panel, and any other parameters deemed necessary by study investigator from baseline after OCU410ST administration.	12 months (Screening to 12 months post-OCU410ST administration)

Other outcome measures

Outcome measure	Measure description	Time frame
Changes in macular thickness on Spectra Domain Optical Coherence Tomography (SD-OCT)	The change in the macular thickness will be measured by spectral domain optical coherence tomography (SD-OCT)	12 months (Screening to 12 months post-OCU410ST administration)
Change in Quality-of-life measure using NEI VFQ-25 (Adult subjects only)	The National Eye Institute Visual Function Questionnaire 25 (NEI-VFQ25) questionnaires will be administered to assess the impact of vision on quality of subject's life.	12 months (Screening to 12 months post-OCU410ST administration)

Sponsor
Ocugen

Collaborators
No information provided

Investigators
- Study Director: Huma Qamar, MD, MPH, CMI, Ocugen., Inc.

General Publications
No publications available

United States

Recruiting

Phase 2 Tolerability and Effects of ALK-001 on Stargardt Disease (TEASE)

ClinicalTrials.gov ID NCT02402660

Sponsor Alkeus Pharmaceuticals, Inc.
Information provided by Alkeus Pharmaceuticals, Inc. (Responsible Party)
Last Update Posted 2022-03-03

More Information
Study Overview

Brief Summary

The purpose of this study is to determine the long-term safety and tolerability of ALK-001 (C20-D3-retinyl acetate) and to explore the effects of ALK-001 on the progression of Stargardt disease in patients between the ages of 8 and 70 years old.

Funding Source – FDA OOPD

Detailed Description

This study evaluates the effects of orally administered ALK-001 on the progression of Stargardt disease (ABCA4-related). Stargardt disease is a rare genetic disorder that leads to damage to the retina and results in legal blindness. Stargardt disease is caused by a defective ABCA4 gene, which affects the processing of vitamin A in the eye and leads to the formation of toxic vitamin A aggregates (called "vitamin A dimers") in the eye. Vitamin A dimers are thought to contribute to vision loss in Stargardt disease. ALK-001, the investigational drug, is a chemically modified vitamin A designed as a replacement of vitamin A to prevent the formation of toxic vitamin A dimers in the eye. Trial participants will receive either ALK-001 or placebo, and follow-up visits will take place periodically for up to 24 months. There is currently no treatment for Stargardt disease.

Official Title

A Phase 2 Multicenter, Double-Masked, Randomized, Placebo-Controlled Study to Investigate the Long-Term Safety, Tolerability, Pharmacokinetics, and Effects of ALK-001 on the Progression of Stargardt Disease

Conditions

Stargardt Disease
Stargardt Macular Degeneration
Stargardt Macular Dystrophy
Autosomal Recessive Stargardt Disease 1 (ABCA4-related)

Intervention/Treatment
- Drug: ALK-001
- Drug: Placebo

Other Study ID Numbers
- ALK001-P1002
- R01FD004098 (U.S. FDA Grant/Contract)
- R01FD006016 (Other Grant/Funding Number) (OTHER_GRANT: FDA OOPD)

Study Start (Actual)
2015-08

Primary Completion (Estimated)
2024-12

Study Completion (Estimated)
2025-03

Enrollment (Estimated)
140

Study Type
Interventional

Phase
Phase 2

Study Contact
Name: Leonide Saad, PhD
Phone Number: 800-287-2755
Email: trials@alkeus.com
United States
California Locations

Los Angeles, California, United States, 90095
Recruiting
University of California Los Angeles – Jules Stein Eye Institute

Principal Investigator
Michael Gorin, MD, PhD

Florida Locations

Gainesville, Florida, United States, 32607
Recruiting
Vitreoretinal Associates

Principal Investigator
Christine Kay, MD

Miami, Florida, United States, 33136
Recruiting
University of Miami – Bascom Palmer Eye Institute

Principal Investigator
Byron Lam, MD

Maryland Locations

Baltimore, Maryland, United States, 21287
Active, not recruiting
Johns Hopkins – Wilmer Eye Institute

New York Locations

New York, New York, United States, 10032
Recruiting
Columbia University Medical Center – Harkness Eye Institute

Principal Investigator
Stephen Tsang, MD, PhD

Utah Locations

Salt Lake City, Utah, United States, 84132
Completed
University of Utah – Moran Eye Institute

Wisconsin Locations

Milwaukee, Wisconsin, United States, 53226
Active, not recruiting
Medical College of Wisconsin – Eye Institute

Eligibility Criteria
Description

Simplified Inclusion Criteria
- Male or female between 8 and 70 years old (inclusive), with any visual acuity
- Has a clinical diagnosis of typical autosomal recessive Stargardt macular dystrophy (STGD1)
- Has provided a genetic report indicating at least two ABCA4 disease-causing mutations. When only one ABCA4 disease-causing mutation is reported, sponsor's permission will be required.
- At least one eye (called the "primary study eye") must have at least one well-demarcated area of significantly reduced autofluorescence as imaged by fundus autofluorescence (FAF), have decreased retinal sensitivity as measured by microperimetry, or have maculopathy expected to progress over the duration of the study

- Primary study eye must have clear ocular media and adequate pupillary dilation, including no allergy to dilating eyedrops, to permit good quality retinal imaging
- Healthy as judged by investigator
- Able and willing to comply with study requirements, restrictions, and instructions and is likely to complete the 24-month study
- Has signed and dated the informed consent forms (or assent where appropriate) to participate
- Female of childbearing potential has signed the informed consent about birth defects or attestation on contraception requirements

Main Exclusion Criteria
- Has taken disallowed items (supplement containing vitamin A or beta-carotene, liver-based products, or prescription oral retinoid medications) over the past 30 days
- Is lactating, pregnant, or has a positive serum or urine pregnancy test at screening or at randomization
- Has concurrent medical condition or history, which in the opinion of the investigator, is likely to prevent compliance with the protocol and/or interfere with absorption of ALK-001 or study procedures
- Has clinically significant abnormal laboratory result(s) at screening
- Has active or historical acute or chronic liver disorder
- Has active or historical ocular disorder in the primary study eye that, in the opinion of the investigator, may confound assessment of the retina morphologically or functionally (this could include, for example, cataract surgery within the past 6 months, choroidal neovascularization (CNV), glaucoma, recurring uveitis, diabetic retinopathy, other retinal disease, etc.)
- Has had intraocular surgery or injections in the primary study eye within 90 days of the screening visit
- Has a clinically significant abnormal electrocardiogram (ECG), or has a corrected QT interval (QTc) that is 450 ms or greater

Ages Eligible for Study
8–70 Years (Child, Adult, Older Adult)

Sexes Eligible for Study
All

Accepts Healthy Volunteers
No

Design Details
Primary Purpose: Treatment
Allocation: Randomized
Interventional Model: Parallel Assignment
Masking: Quadruple (Participant Care Provider Investigator Outcomes Assessor)

Arms and interventions

Participant group/arm	Intervention/treatment

Experimental: ALK-001
Daily, oral administration of one capsule. See details below.
	Drug: ALK-001
	• Daily, oral administration for 24 months
	• Other Names:
	   – C20-D3-Retinyl Acetate
	   – C20 Deuterated vitamin A

Placebo Comparator: Placebo Daily, oral administration of one capsule. See details below.	Drug: Placebo • Daily, oral administration for 24 months

Primary outcome measures

Outcome measure	Measure description	Time frame
Safety and tolerability of 24 months of daily dosing of ALK-001 assessed by Incidence and/or clinically significant changes of a combination of ocular and non-ocular adverse events		From baseline to 24 months

Secondary outcome measures

Outcome measure	Measure description	Time frame
Effects of ALK-001 on the progression of Stargardt disease	Combination of changes in atrophic lesion size, best-corrected visual acuity (BCVA), and ocular assessments.	From baseline to 24 months
Pharmacokinetic profile of ALK-001 derived from the concentrations of ALK-001 and metabolites in plasma		Up to 24 months

Sponsor

Alkeus Pharmaceuticals, Inc.

Collaborators

No information provided

Investigators

• Study Director: Hendrik Scholl, MD, University of Basel
• Study Director: Leonide Saad, PhD, Alkeus Pharmaceuticals, Inc.

General Publications

• Ma L, Kaufman Y, Zhang J, Washington I. C20-D3-vitamin A slows lipofuscin accumulation and electrophysiological retinal degeneration in a mouse model of Stargardt disease. J Biol Chem. 2011 Mar 11;286(10):7966–7974. https://doi.org/10.1074/jbc.M110.178657. Epub 2010 Dec 14.

- Kaufman Y, Ma L, Washington I. Deuterium enrichment of vitamin A at the C20 position slows the formation of detrimental vitamin A dimers in wild-type rodents. J Biol Chem. 2011 Mar 11;286(10):7958–7965. https://doi.org/10.1074/jbc.M110.178640. Epub 2010 Nov 12.
- Mihai DM, Jiang H, Blaner WS, Romanov A, Washington I. The retina rapidly incorporates ingested C20-D(3)-vitamin A in a swine model. Mol Vis. 2013 Jul 25;19:1677–83. Print 2013.
- Charbel Issa P, Barnard AR, Herrmann P, Washington I, MacLaren RE. Rescue of the Stargardt phenotype in Abca4 knockout mice through inhibition of vitamin A dimerization. Proc Natl Acad Sci U S A. 2015 Jul 7;112(27):8415–20. https://doi.org/10.1073/pnas.1506960112. Epub 2015 Jun 23.
- Saad L, Washington I. Can Vitamin A be Improved to Prevent Blindness due to Age-Related Macular Degeneration, Stargardt Disease and Other Retinal Dystrophies? Adv Exp Med Biol. 2016;854:355–61. https://doi.org/10.1007/978-3-319-17121-0_47.
- Zhang D, Robinson K, Washington I. C20D3-Vitamin A Prevents Retinal Pigment Epithelium Atrophic Changes in a Mouse Model. Transl Vis Sci Technol. 2021 Dec 1;10(14):8. https://doi.org/10.1167/tvst.10.14.8.
- Zhang D, Robinson K, Saad L, Washington I. Vitamin A cycle byproducts impede dark adaptation. J Biol Chem. 2021 Sep;297(3):101074. https://doi.org/10.1016/j.jbc.2021.101074. Epub 2021 Aug 12.

United States

Recruiting

Rod- and Cone-Mediated Function in Retinal Disease

ClinicalTrials.gov ID NCT02617966

Sponsor National Eye Institute (NEI)
Information provided by National Institutes of Health Clinical Center (CC) (National Eye Institute (NEI)) (Responsible Party)
Last Update Posted 2023-10-17

Study Overview

Brief Summary
Background
Retinal diseases cause the loss of rod and cone photoreceptors. Symptoms include vision loss and night blindness. Researchers want to learn about rod and cone function in healthy people and people with retinal disease. They want to know if how well a person sees in the dark can test the severity of retinal disease.

Objectives

To find out if how well a person sees in the dark can test the severity of retinal disease. To find out if this can help detect retinal disease and track its changes.

Eligibility

People aged 5 and older with:

Retinal Disease OR

20/20 vision or better with or without correction in at least one eye

Design
- Participants will be screened with medical and eye history and eye exam. Those with retinal disease will also have:
- Eye imaging: Drops dilate the eye and pictures are taken of it.
- Visual field testing: Participants look into a bowl and press a button when they see light.
- Electroretinogram (ERG): An electrode is taped to the forehead. Participants sit in the dark with their eyes patched for 30 min. Then they get numbing drops and contact lenses. Participants watch lights while retina signals are recorded.
- Visit 1 will be 3–8 h. Participants will have up to 6 more visits over 6–12 months. Visits include:

Eye Exam and Imaging
- Time course of dark adaptation: Participants view a background light for 5 min, then push a button when they see colored light.
- Dark adapted sensitivity: Participants sit in the dark for 45 min. They push a button when they see colored light.
- For participants with retinal disease, ERG and visual field testing

Detailed Description
- Objective: The objective of this protocol is to investigate local changes in rod and cone photoreceptor function across the retina in healthy volunteers and participants with retinal disease.
- Study Population: Up to 120 healthy volunteers and 250 participants, aged five or older, with retinal disease.
- Design: This single-center, observational, case-control study will be comprised of three related Aims that assess rod and cone function with the recently released commercial Medmont Dark Adapted Chromatic (DAC) perimeter and/or a commercial Cambridge Research Systems computer monitor (Display++) specialized for displaying stimuli at low light intensities and/or the scotopic MP1S perimeter.
- For Aim 1, the normal ranges will be established for dark-adapted retinal sensitivities to blue and red stimuli of the DAC perimeter, and MP1S perimeter, and for radial frequency (RF) hyperacuity on the Display++ monitor. For Aim 2, the normal range will be established for describing the kinetics of dark adaptation following bleaching of retinal rhodopsin for the DAC and MP1S perimeters. For

Aim 3, local changes in rod and cone photoreceptor function across the retina in participants with retinal disease will be examined from measurement of the kinetics of dark adaptation, dark-adapted retinal sensitivity to the DAC blue and red stimuli, and/or RF hyperacuity on the Display++ monitor, and/or the MP1S perimeter.

- Outcome Measures: The primary outcome for this study is to establish normal ranges for (A) the kinetics of dark adaptation (time), (B) dark-adapted retinal sensitivity (dB) for the Medmont DAC and MP1S blue and red stimuli, and C) RF hyperacuity on the Display++ monitor. The secondary outcomes will be to examine changes in the kinetics of dark adaptation, dark-adapted retinal sensitivity, and scotopic and photopic RF hyperacuity in participants with retinal disease.

Official Title
Rod- and Cone-Mediated Function in Retinal Disease

Conditions
Retinal Degeneration
Retinitis Pigmentosa
Stargardt Disease

Intervention/Treatment

Other Study ID Numbers
- 160024
- 16-EI-0024

Study Start (Actual)
2016-03-24

Primary Completion (Estimated)
2029-12-30

Study Completion (Estimated)
2029-12-30

Enrollment (Estimated)
370
Study Type
Observational

Study Contact
Name: Daniel W Claus, R.N.
Phone Number: (301) 451-1621
Email: daniel.claus@nih.gov
Study Contact Backup
Name: Brett G Jeffrey, Ph.D.
Phone Number: (301) 402-2391
Email: jeffreybg@mail.nih.gov

United States
Maryland Locations

Bethesda, Maryland, United States, 20892
Recruiting
National Institutes of Health Clinical Center

Eligibility Criteria
Description

Inclusion Criteria
- Participant must be 5 years of age or older.
- Participant (or legal guardian) must understand and sign the protocol's informed consent document.
- Participant must be able to cooperate with the testing required for this study.

For Participants with Retinal Disease Only
- Participant must have retinal disease, defined as evidence of loss of retinal dysfunction and/or degeneration as established by standard clinical methods including perimetry, ERG, and imaging.
- Participant must have a measurable visual acuity.

For Healthy Volunteers Only
- Participant must have visual acuity of 20/20 or better, with or without correction (e.g., glasses or contact lens), in at least one eye.

Exclusion Criteria
- Participant with changes in pre-retinal media sufficient to obscure a view of the retina.

Show less
Study Population
Up to 250 participants with retinal disease will be enrolled and up to 120 healthy volunteers will be enrolled.

Ages Eligible for Study
5 Years to 100 Years (Child, Adult, Older Adult)

Sexes Eligible for Study
All

Accepts Healthy Volunteers
Yes
Sampling Method
Non-Probability Sample

Design Details
Observational Model: Case-Control
Time Perspective: Cross-Sectional

Cohorts and interventions

Group/cohort
Affected Participants with retinal disease
Unaffected Healthy volunteers

Primary outcome measures

Outcome measure	Measure description	Time frame
The primary outcomes for this study are to establish normal ranges for the kinetics of dark adaptation and dark-adapted retinal sensitivity for the fundus-guided and non-guided perimeters and for RF hyperacuity on the Display++.	The primary outcomes for this study are to establish normal ranges for the kinetics of dark adaptation and dark-adapted retinal sensitivity for the fundus-guided and non-guided perimeters and for RF hyperacuity on the Display++.	ongoing, up to 10 visits in 5 years

Secondary outcome measures

Outcome measure	Measure description	Time frame
Secondary outcomes will be to examine changes in the kinetics of dark adaptation and dark-adapted retinal sensitivity, and scotopic and photopic RF hyperacuity in participants with retinal disease.	Secondary outcomes will be to examine changes in the kinetics of dark adaptation and dark-adapted retinal sensitivity, and scotopic and photopic RF hyperacuity in participants with retinal disease.	ongoing, up to four visits in 5 years

Sponsor
National Eye Institute (NEI)

Collaborators
No information provided

Investigators
- Principal Investigator: Brett G Jeffrey, Ph.D., National Eye Institute (NEI)

General Publications
- Jackson GR, Owsley C, Curcio CA. Photoreceptor degeneration and dysfunction in aging and age-related maculopathy. Ageing Res Rev. 2002 Jun;1(3):381–96. https://doi.org/10.1016/s1568-1637(02)00007-7.
- Massof RW, Finkelstein D. Rod sensitivity relative to cone sensitivity in retinitis pigmentosa. Invest Ophthalmol Vis Sci. 1979 Mar;18(3):263–72.
- Birch DG, Wen Y, Locke K, Hood DC. Rod sensitivity, cone sensitivity, and photoreceptor layer thickness in retinal degenerative diseases. Invest Ophthalmol Vis Sci. 2011 Sep 9;52(10):7141–7. https://doi.org/10.1167/iovs.11-7509.

United States

Recruiting

Stargardt-Like Macular Dystrophy (STDG3) Secondary to Mutations in ELOVL4

ClinicalTrials.gov ID NCT04591483

Sponsor National Eye Institute (NEI)
Information provided by National Institutes of Health Clinical Center (CC) (National Eye Institute (NEI)) (Responsible Party)
Last Update Posted 2023-10-16

Study Overview

Brief Summary
Background
STDG3 is an inherited eye disease. Currently there is no treatment for STDG3. Past studies of STDG3 have largely looked at members of large families at a single time point. Researchers want to learn more about the disease at an individual level.

Objective
To understand the natural history of changes in the retina that occur in people with STDG3.

Eligibility
People age 10 and older with STDG3 due to a variant in the ELOVL4 gene.

Design
Participants will have 6 visits. First, they will have a screening visit, followed by a baseline visit. Then they will have a visit 6 months later. Then they will have a visit 1, 2, and 3 years after the first visit. Visits will last 4–8 h.
Visits will include the following:

Medical history and physical exam.
Complete eye exam. Participants' eye pressure and ability to see letters on a vision chart will be tested. Their pupils will be dilated with eye drops. Pictures will be taken of the retina and the inside of the eye.
Questions about participants' family history, especially the presence of eye disease.
Visual field test. Participants will be seated in front of a large dome and asked to press a button when they see a light within the dome.
Electroretinogram. Participants will sit in the dark with their eyes patched for 30 min. Then they will wear special contact lenses and watch flashing lights.

Optical coherence tomography. Cross-sectional pictures will be taken of participants' retinas.

Fundus autofluorescence. Blue light will be shone into participants' eyes to assess the health of the retina.

Detailed Description

Title: An Observational Prospective Natural History Study of Stargardt-like Macular Dystrophy (STDG3) Secondary to Mutations in ELOVL4

Study Description: Potential therapeutics for Stargardt-like macular dystrophy (STDG3) have been proposed. Cross-sectional studies of large families suggest progressive macular atrophy in STDG3, but there is a paucity of longitudinal data for these patients. The overall goal is to establish a natural history study of STDG3.

Objectives: The primary objective is to assess the longitudinal changes in retinal structure in STDG3 patients.

The secondary objective is to assess the longitudinal changes in retinal function in STDG3 patients.

An exploratory objective is to assess the longitudinal changes in functional vision and the participant's perceived effect on activities of daily living (e.g., mobility).

Endpoints: The primary endpoints are: A) the growth rate of the square root area of loss of the inner segment/outer segment band (EZband) obtained from spectral-domain optical coherence tomography (SD-OCT) and B) the rate of atrophy enlargement obtained from fundus autofluorescence.

The secondary endpoints are: (A) the change in BCVA total letters read from baseline to Year 3 and (B) the rate of loss of retinal sensitivity measured with perimetry.

Study Population: Up to 25 patients with Stargardt-like macular dystrophy 3 who are >= 10 years of age.

Description of Sites/Facilities Enrolling Participants: Patients will be seen in the Ophthalmic Genetics Clinic at the National Eye Institute within the NIH Clinical Center in Bethesda.

Study Duration: 84 months (7 years).

Participant Duration: 36 months (3 years).

Official Title

An Observational Prospective Natural History Study of Stargardt-like Macular Dystrophy (STDG3) Secondary to Mutations in ELOVL4

Conditions

Stargardt-Like Macular Dystrophy

Intervention/Treatment

Other Study ID Numbers

- 10000108
- 000108-EI

Study Start (Actual)
2022-04-19

Primary Completion (Estimated)
2028-07-16

Study Completion (Estimated)
2028-07-16

Enrollment (Estimated)
25

Study Type
Observational

Study Contact
Name: Daniel W Claus, R.N.
Phone Number: (301) 451-1621
Email: daniel.claus@nih.gov
Study Contact Backup
Name: Brett G Jeffrey, Ph.D.
Phone Number: (301) 402-2391
Email: jeffreybg@mail.nih.gov

United States
Maryland Locations

Bethesda, Maryland, United States, 20892
Recruiting
National Institutes of Health Clinical Center

Contact
For more information at the NIH Clinical Center, contact Office of Patient
   Recruitment (OPR)
800-411-1222 ext TTY8664111010 prpl@cc.nih.gov

Eligibility Criteria
Description

Inclusion Criteria
To be eligible, the following inclusion criteria must be met, where applicable.

- Stated willingness to comply with all study procedures and availability for the
  duration of the study.
- Participant must be at least ten years of age.
- Ability to perform required functional testing and ophthalmic imaging.
- A mutation in ELOVL4 with a typical clinical presentation of Stargardt-like
  macular dystrophy.
- Participant (or legal guardian) must understand and sign the protocol' s informed
  consent document.

Exclusion Criteria

A participant is not eligible if any of the following exclusion criteria are present.

- Two or more definitive mutations in ABCA4 and/or one mutation in RDS/peripherin or PROM1.
- Systemic medical contraindications that are rarely associated with ELOVL4 (e.g., Spinocerebellar Ataxia-34).

Study Population

Twenty-five patients with Stargardt-like macular dystrophy 3 who are >= 10 years of age.

Ages Eligible for Study

10–100 Years (Child, Adult, Older Adult)

Sexes Eligible for Study

All

Accepts Healthy Volunteers

No
Sampling Method
Non-Probability Sample

Design Details

Observational Model: Cohort
Time Perspective: Prospective

Cohorts and interventions

Group/cohort
Affected
Patients with Stargardt-like macular dystrophy 3 who are >= 10 years of age.

Primary outcome measures

Outcome measure	Measure description	Time frame
Growth rate in square root area of loss of the inner segment/outer segment band (band)	The growth rate of the square root area of loss of the inner segment/outer segment band (band) obtained from SD-OCT.	Day 1, 182, 364, 728, 1,092
Growth rate of square root area of atrophy measured from short-wavelength autofluorescence	The rate of atrophy enlargement obtained from fundus autofluorescence.	Day 1, 182, 364, 728, 1,092

Secondary outcome measures

Outcome measure	Measure description	Time frame
The change in BCVA total letters read from baseline to Year 3	The change in BCVA total letters read from baseline to Year 3.	Day 1, 182, 364, 728, 1,092

Outcome measure	Measure description	Time frame
The rate of loss of retinal sensitivity measured with perimetry	The rate of loss of retinal sensitivity measured with perimetry.	Day 1, 182, 364, 728, 1,092

Sponsor
National Eye Institute (NEI)

Collaborators
National Cancer Institute (NCI)

Investigators
- Principal Investigator: Brett G Jeffrey, Ph.D., National Eye Institute (NEI)

General Publications
No publications available

United States

Recruiting

Oral Metformin for Treatment of ABCA4 Retinopathy

ClinicalTrials.gov ID NCT04545736

Sponsor National Eye Institute (NEI)
Information provided by National Institutes of Health Clinical Center (CC) (National Eye Institute (NEI)) (Responsible Party)
Last Update Posted 2023-08-24

Study Overview

Brief Summary
Background
ABCA4 retinopathy is a genetic disease in which the ABCA4 protein is absent or faulty. It can cause waste material to collect in the eye and may cause cells to die. The cell death can lead to vision loss. Researchers want to see if an oral drug called metformin can help.

Objective
To see if metformin is safe and possibly helps to slow the rate of ABCA4 retinopathy.

Eligibility
People aged 12 and older who have ABCA4 retinopathy and have problems with their vision.

Design

Participants will be screened under a separate protocol.

Participants will have a medical and family history. They will complete a questionnaire about their vision and daily activities. They will have a physical exam. They may have blood drawn through a needle in the arm.

Participants will have an eye exam. Their pupils may be dilated with eye drops. Their retina may be photographed.

Participants will have a visual field test. They will sit in front of a large dome and press a button when they see a light within the dome.

Participants will have an electroretinogram. It examines the function of the retina. They will sit in the dark for 30 min. Then their eyes will be numbed with eye drops. They will wear contact lenses that can sense signals from the retinas. They will watch flashing lights.

Participants will have optical coherence tomography. This noninvasive procedure makes pictures of the retina.

Participants will have fundus autofluorescence. A bright blue light will be shone into their eye.

Participants will take metformin by mouth for 24 months.

Participants will have study visits every 6 months. Participation will last for at least 36 months....

Detailed Description

Study Description

ABCA4 retinopathy is an autosomal recessive progressive retinal dystrophy that leads to retinal pigment epithelium (RPE) and photoreceptor degeneration, with consequent central visual loss. A treatment that either reduces the rate of lipofuscin accumulation or improves the clearance of lipofuscin in the RPE which could potentially slow the degeneration associated with this disease. Metformin hydrochloride is a well-characterized, commonly prescribed oral antidiabetic medication that acts by suppressing liver gluconeogenesis and increasing peripheral insulin sensitivity.

An additional effect of metformin is to increase macroautophagy via the Mammalian target of rapamycin complex 1 (mTORC1)/AMP-activated Kinase (AMPK) pathway; stimulation of this pathway would be predicted to enable the RPE to more efficiently handle lipofuscin. This suggests an association between metformin use and slowing of retinal degeneration. The objective of this study is to investigate the safety and potential efficacy of oral metformin in slowing the rate of change in photoreceptor degeneration in ABCA4 retinopathy.

Objectives

The objective of this study is to investigate the safety and potential efficacy of oral metformin in slowing the rate of change in photoreceptor degeneration in ABCA4 retinopathy.

Endpoints

Primary Endpoint: The difference in growth rate of square-root-transformed area of EZ band loss (square-root Area loss), from OCT, between the pretreatment phase and 24 month metformin treatment phase.

Secondary Endpoints: Proportion of participants with a 30% reduction in growth rate of square-root area loss during the treatment phase compared to the pretreatment phase, changes from baseline to Month 24 in Best-Corrected Visual Acuity (BCVA) total letters read, perimetry, and color fundus photography measurements and the change in rate of area of atrophy enlargement between the pretreatment and 24-month metformin treatment phase.

Official Title

Oral Metformin for Treatment of ABCA4 Retinopathy

Conditions

ABCA4 Retinopathy
Stargardt Disease
Retinal Dystrophy
Retinal Degeneration

Intervention/Treatment

- Drug: Metformin hydrochloride

Other Study ID Numbers

- 200163
- 20-EI-0163

Study Start (Actual)

2020-11-23

Primary Completion (Estimated)

2027-08-31

Study Completion (Estimated)

2027-08-31

Enrollment (Estimated)

45

Study Type

Interventional

Phase

Phase 1 and Phase 2

Study Contact

Name: Cathy Kangale-Whitney, R.N.
Phone Number: (301) 402-4174
Email: cathy.kangale-whitney@nih.gov
Study Contact Backup
Name: Brian P Brooks, M.D.

Phone Number: (301) 496-3577
Email: brooksb@mail.nih.gov
United States
Maryland Locations

Bethesda, Maryland, United States, 20892
Recruiting
National Institutes of Health Clinical Center

Contact
For more information at the NIH Clinical Center contact Office of Patient
   Recruitment (OPR)
800-411-1222 ext TTY8664111010 prpl@cc.nih.gov

Michigan Locations

Ann Arbor, Michigan, United States, 48109-0624
Recruiting
University of Michigan

Contact
Abby Sharp
734-232-9594 abmckee@med.umich.edu

Eligibility Criteria
Description

Inclusion Criteria
To be eligible, the following inclusion criteria must be met, where applicable.

- Participant must be at least 12 years of age.
- Participant (or legal guardian) must understand and sign the protocol's
  informed consent document.
- Participant must have at least one definite pathogenic or likely pathogenic
  mutation in ABCA4 and a typical clinical presentation of Stargardt disease
  and phenotypic presentation of ABCA4 retinopathy in both eyes.
- Participant must have at least two years of natural history data from at least
  four data points (a). The separation between any two consecutive data points
  must be at least six months (b). The most recent data point must be at least 4.5
  months and no more than 16 months prior to the baseline visit (c).

  - Potential participants with three natural history data points may be enrolled
    to obtain their fourth natural history data point on protocol.
  - The separation between any two consecutive data points may fall short of
    6 months by no more than 45 days; however, the total separation among
    the data points must allow for at least two years of natural history data.
  - Potential participants with four or more natural history data points com-
    pleted off protocol, all of which having occurred more than 16 months
    prior to the baseline visit, may be enrolled to complete an additional natu-
    ral history data point on protocol within the required timeframe from the
    baseline visit.

- Participant must agree to adhere to Lifestyle Considerations throughout study duration.
- Any female participant of childbearing potential must have a negative urine pregnancy test at screening and be willing to undergo urine pregnancy tests throughout the study.
- Female participant of childbearing potential and male participants or their partners must have (or have a partner who has) had a surgical sterilization (vasectomy, hysterectomy, or tubal ligation), be completely abstinent from intercourse, or must agree to practice at least one acceptable method of contraception throughout the course of the study and for at least one week after IP discontinuation for female participants or for at least 3 months after IP discontinuation for male participants or their partners. Acceptable methods of contraception include:

  – hormonal contraception (i.e., birth control pills, injected hormones, dermal patch, or vaginal ring),
  – intrauterine device,
  – barrier methods (diaphragm, condom) with spermicide.

  Metformin, like insulin, is considered a class B drug by the FDA (animal reproductive studies have failed to demonstrate a risk to the fetus and there are no adequate and well-controlled studies in pregnant women) and is frequently prescribed for gestational diabetes. One meta-analysis showed outcomes with metformin were slightly superior to insulin. Nonetheless, out of an abundance of caution, we will ask female and male participants in this trial to use these forms of contraception.

Exclusion Criteria

An individual who meets any of the following criteria will be excluded from participation in this study:

- Participant is actively receiving study IP in another investigational study.
- Participant has a condition that would preclude participation in the study (e.g., unstable medical status including blood pressure and glycemic control) by interfering with the participant's ability to engage in the required protocol evaluation and testing and/or comply with study visits.
- Any female participant of childbearing potential who is pregnant, breast-feeding, or planning to become pregnant during the study.
- Participant has definitive mutations in RDS/peripherin (PRPH2), PROM1, and/or ELOVL4.
- Participant has a history of chronic renal impairment as measured in the acute care panel-estimated glomerular filtration rate (eGFR<45 ml/min/1.73 m2) or severe hepatic, pulmonary, or cardiovascular disease (hypoxic state).
- Participant is taking any medication that could adversely interact with metformin (e.g., cimetidine, furosemide, nifedipine) and cannot switch to an alternative medication.
- Participant is currently taking metformin or participant has taken metformin during the period of natural history data collection that will be used for this study for a cumulative total of more than one month.

- Participant has a known hypersensitivity to metformin.
- Participant has a history of chronic lactic acidosis, including diabetic ketoacidosis, with or without coma.
- Participant has type 1 diabetes mellitus.
- Scarring due to choroidal neovascularization (CNV) is present in either eye.

Qualifying Eye Eligibility Criteria

In order to participate in the study, the participant must have at least one qualifying eye that meets all of the inclusion and none of the exclusion criteria listed below.

Qualifying Eye Inclusion Criteria

1. A growth rate of square-root Area loss > 0.025 mm/year based on calculation from natural history data.

Qualifying Eye Exclusion Criteria

1. Retinal degeneration has advanced beyond a point where reliable measurement of the integrity of the IS-OS on OCT is possible.

Ages Eligible for Study

12–100 Years (Child, Adult, Older Adult)

Sexes Eligible for Study

All

Accepts Healthy Volunteers

No

Design Details

Primary Purpose: Treatment
Allocation: N/A
Interventional Model: Single Group Assignment
Masking: None (Open Label)

Arms and interventions

Participant group/arm	Intervention/treatment
Experimental: Metformin Oral administration of metformin	Drug: Metformin hydrochloride • Metformin is commercially produced in immediate and extended release. Participants will receive an immediate release formulation of metformin of 500 mg daily at study entry. This dose will be titrated up weekly in 500 mg increments to reach a goal of 2000 mg daily maximum. Once participants >=17 years of age reach 2000 mg metformin immediate release, they will switch to an extended-release formulation (1000 mg twice a day by mouth). Participants >= 17 years of age who cannot tolerate 2000 mg will be permitted to reduce their daily dose to a minimum of 1000mg/day. Because metformin extended release is not FDA-approved for children under the age of 17, participants under 17 will remain on the immediate release formulation. For these participants who remain on standard formulation, the maximum tolerated dose between 1000 mg and 2000 mg/day will be given.

Primary outcome measures

Outcome measure	Measure description	Time frame
The difference in growth rate of square-root-transformed area of band loss (Area loss)	The difference in growth rate of area loss, from OCT, between the pretreatment phase and treatment phase.	Pretreatment, Baseline, Month 24

Secondary outcome measures

Outcome measure	Measure description	Time frame
Proportion of participants with a 30% reduction in growth rate of area loss	Proportion of participants with 30% reduction in growth rate of area loss, from OCT, during the treatment phase compared to the pretreatment phase.	Pretreatment, Baseline, Month 24
Number and severity of adverse events	The number and severity of systemic and ocular toxicities, adverse events and infections by severity, type and assessed relatedness to the IP throughout the study period.	ongoing throughout study
Changes in best-corrected visual acuity (BCVA)	The change in BCVA total letters read from baseline to Month 24.	Baseline, Month 24
Change in rate of area of atrophy enlargement	The difference in rate of region of atrophy measurements from FAF between the pretreatment phase and treatment phase.	Pretreatment, Baseline, Month 24
Change in perimetry and color fundus photography measurements	The change in perimetry and color fundus photography from baseline to Month 24.	Baseline, Month 24

Sponsor
National Eye Institute (NEI)

Collaborators
No information provided

Investigators
- Principal Investigator: Brian P Brooks, M.D., National Eye Institute (NEI)

General Publications
No publications available

United States

Recruiting

Genotype-Phenotype Study of Patients with Plaquenil-Induced Retinal Toxicity, with Evaluation of the ABCA4 Gene

ClinicalTrials.gov ID NCT01145196

Sponsor National Eye Institute (NEI)
Information provided by National Institutes of Health Clinical Center (CC) (National Eye Institute (NEI)) (Responsible Party)
Last Update Posted 2023-10-23

Study Overview

Brief Summary
Background
– Plaquenil (hydroxychloroquine) is an anti-inflammatory drug that is used to treat some autoimmune diseases such as lupus and rheumatoid arthritis. This drug can damage the retina by causing a condition called plaquenil-induced retinal toxicity, which may lead to vision loss. However, most people taking plaquenil do not develop this problem. Researchers are interested in studying whether differences in a person's genes explain why some people develop plaquenil-induced retinal toxicity while others do not.

Objectives
– To investigate possible correlations between certain genes or genetic mutations and plaquenil-induced retinal toxicity.

Eligibility
• Individuals at least 18 years of age who have previously used plaquenil.
• Both individuals who have and have not developed plaquenil-induced retinal toxicity will be eligible for this study.

Design
• The study requires one or two visits to the National Eye Institute or an outpatient study clinic over a maximum 2-year period.
• Participants will provide a personal and family medical history and will have a full eye examination.
• Participants will also provide blood samples for testing.
• No treatment will be provided as part of this protocol.

Detailed Description
Objective
The objective of this study is to investigate whether there is a correlation between genetic mutations, beginning with an analysis of ABCA4, and Plaquenil-induced retinal toxicity and to describe the phenotype of Plaquenil-induced retinal toxicity.

Study Population
The study will enroll 100 patients, 18 years of age or older, found to have Plaquenil-induced retinal toxicity. Two hundred volunteers with systemic lupus erythematosus (SLE), rheumatoid arthritis (RA), or Sjogren's syndrome and history of Plaquenil use, but without evidence of retinal toxicity, will also be recruited.

Design
The study is an observational study with 1–2 outpatient visits to the NEI clinic or review of medical records for off-site participants. All participants will provide a blood sample for genetic analysis.

Outcome Measures
Clinical examination and blood samples will be used for genetic testing and mutation identification. The primary outcome of this study is to identify genetic mutations, starting with those in ABCA4 gene, associated with retinal toxicity in participants with a history of Plaquenil use. Secondary objectives include determining the utility of testing metrics in evaluating the presence of retinal toxicity.

Official Title
Genotype – Phenotype Study of Patients With Plaquenil-induced Retinal Toxicity

Conditions
Genotype
Retinal Disease

Intervention/Treatment

Other Study ID Numbers
- 100140
- 10-EI-0140

Study Start (Actual)
2010-08-23

Primary Completion
Study Completion

Enrollment (Estimated)
300

Study Type
Observational

Study Contact

Name: Faith Chen
Phone Number: (301) 402-1369
Email: chenfa@nei.nih.gov
Study Contact Backup
Name: Emily Y Chew, M.D.
Phone Number: (301) 496-6583
Email: echew@nei.nih.gov
United States
Maryland Locations

Bethesda, Maryland, United States, 20892
Recruiting
National Institutes of Health Clinical Center

Contact

For more information at the NIH Clinical Center contact Office of Patient
Recruitment (OPR)
800-411-1222 ext TTY dial 711 ccopr@nih.gov

Eligibility Criteria
Description

Inclusion Criteria

- Affected participants must be 18 years of age or older and have:

  - History of systemic lupus erythematosus (SLE), rheumatoid arthritis (RA), or
    Sjogren's syndrome, and
  - History of Plaquenil use, and
  - Evidence of Plaquenil-induced retinal toxicity, based on clinical findings.

- Unaffected volunteers must be 18 years of age or older and have:

  - History of systemic lupus erythematosus (SLE), rheumatoid arthritis (RA), or
    Sj (SqrRoot)(Delta)gren s syndrome, and
  - History of Plaquenil use, and
  - No retinal disease upon examination within the last six months.

- All participants must be able to:

  - Provide their own consent, and
  - Safely provide a blood sample.

Exclusion Criteria

- Participants with other known (genetic) retinal disease including but not limited
  to: Stargardt's disease and cone or cone-rod dystrophy whose diagnosis preceded
  their Plaquenil use. Participants with no known previous genetic diagnosis but
  with clinical findings associated with a genetic diagnosis, such as parafoveal or
  macular flecks which are associated with Stargardt's disease or fundus flavimaculatus, will also be excluded.

Study Population

The study will enroll 100 patients, 18 years of age or older, found to have Plaquenil-induced retinal toxicity. Two hundred volunteers with systemic lupus erythematosus (SLE), rheumatoid arthritis (RA), or Sjogren's syndrome and history of Plaquenil use, but without evidence of retinal toxicity, will also be recruited.

Ages Eligible for Study

18 Years and older (Adult, Older Adult)

Sexes Eligible for Study

All

Accepts Healthy Volunteers

No

Sampling Method

Non-Probability Sample

Design Details

Observational Model: Cohort

Time Perspective: Cross-Sectional

Cohorts and interventions

Group/cohort
Affected
Participants affected by Plaquenil-induced retinal toxicity
Unaffected
control participants without Plaquenil-induced retinal toxicity

Primary outcome measures

Outcome measure	Measure description	Time frame
The outcome of this study is to identify genetic mutations, starting with those in ABCA4 gene, associated with retinal toxicity in participants with a history of plaquenil use.	The outcome of this study is to identify genetic mutations, starting with those in ABCA4 gene, associated with retinal toxicity in participants with a history of plaquenil use.	annually for five years

Secondary outcome measures

Outcome measure	Measure description	Time frame
The secondary outcome of this study is to determine the utility of various testing metrics in evaluating the presence of retinal toxicity.	The secondary outcome of this study is to determine the utility of various testing metrics in evaluating the presence of retinal toxicity.	annually for 5 years

Sponsor

National Eye Institute (NEI)

Collaborators
No information provided

Investigators
- Principal Investigator: Emily Y Chew, M.D., National Eye Institute (NEI)

General Publications
- Levy GD, Munz SJ, Paschal J, Cohen HB, Pince KJ, Peterson T. Incidence of hydroxychloroquine retinopathy in 1,207 patients in a large multicenter outpatient practice. Arthritis Rheum. 1997 Aug;40(8):1482–6. https://doi.org/10.1002/art.1780400817.
- HOBBS HE, SORSBY A, FREEDMAN A. Retinopathy following chloroquine therapy. Lancet. 1959 Oct 3;2(7101):478–80. https://doi.org/10.1016/s0140-6736(59)90604-x. No abstract available.
- Webster AR, Heon E, Lotery AJ, Vandenburgh K, Casavant TL, Oh KT, Beck G, Fishman GA, Lam BL, Levin A, Heckenlively JR, Jacobson SG, Weleber RG, Sheffield VC, Stone EM. An analysis of allelic variation in the ABCA4 gene. Invest Ophthalmol Vis Sci. 2001 May;42(6):1179–89.

United States

Recruiting

Inherited Retinal Degenerative Disease Registry (MRTR)

ClinicalTrials.gov ID NCT02435940

Sponsor Foundation Fighting Blindness
Information provided by Foundation Fighting Blindness (Responsible Party)
Last Update Posted 2023-02-15

Study Overview

Brief Summary
The My Retina Tracker® Registry is sponsored by the Foundation Fighting Blindness and is for people affected by one of the rare inherited retinal degenerative diseases studied by the Foundation. It is a patient-initiated registry accessible via a secure online portal at www.MyRetinaTracker.org. Affected individuals who register are guided to create a profile that captures their perspective on their retinal disease and its progress; family history; genetic testing results; preventive measures; general health and interest in participation in research studies. The participants may also choose to ask their clinician to add clinical measurements and results at each clinical visit. Participants are urged to update the information regularly to create longitudinal records of their disease, from their own perspective, and their clinical progress. The overall goals of the Registry are: to better understand the diversity

within the inherited retinal degenerative diseases; to understand the prevalence of the different diseases and gene variants; to assist in the establishment of genotype-phenotype relationships; to help understand the natural history of the diseases; to help accelerate research and development of clinical trials for treatments; and to provide a tool to investigators that can assist with recruitment for research studies and clinical trials.

Detailed Description

My Retina Tracker Registry provides two portals for data entry and review. Initial registration in the My Retina Tracker Registry is initiated by a participant, not a clinician. Using the participant portal, the participant establishes a username and password, is guided through online informed consent, and can then use an interactive guide to record their ophthalmic and family history, genotype and other subjective diagnosis-related and general health information. Drop-down menus and standardized vocabulary are used for database consistency. They may also attach documents, such as medical records, to maintain their personal medical files on their disease. Participants are encouraged to update their profiles regularly to create a longitudinal history of their disease. Participants can see aggregated data for all other participants in the registry and compare their own disease and status to others.

After a profile has been established, Registry members may ask their clinician or genetic counselor to add specific ophthalmic exam and measurement results to the profile. This is done through the clinical portal which also uses a series of drop-down menus to expedite entry and standardize data. Clinicians cannot see the participant data when adding the clinical exam data. Participants are encouraged to collect these data at each medical exam, to create a longitudinal clinical data set.

Access to de-identified data or study recruitment assistance is available to qualified investigators who may inquire by contacting Coordinator@MyRetinaTracker. org. A process that maintains patient anonymity and privacy protection exists for researchers with Institutional Review Board-approved projects who wish to contact registry participants of interest.

Official Title

Foundation Fighting Blindness My Retina Tracker Registry

Conditions

Eye Diseases Hereditary
Retinal Disease
Achromatopsia
Bardet-Biedl Syndrome
Bassen-Kornzweig Syndrome
Batten Disease
Best Disease
Choroidal Dystrophy
Choroideremia
Cone Dystrophy
Cone-Rod Dystrophy

Congenital Stationary Night Blindness
Enhanced S-Cone Syndrome
Fundus Albipunctatus
Goldmann-Favre Syndrome
Gyrate Atrophy
Juvenile Macular Degeneration
Kearns-Sayre Syndrome
Leber Congenital Amaurosis
Refsum Syndrome
Retinitis Pigmentosa
Retinitis Punctata Albescens
Retinoschisis
Rod-Cone Dystrophy
Rod Dystrophy
Rod Monochromacy
Stargardt Disease
Usher Syndrome
Show fewer conditions

Intervention/Treatment

Other Study ID Numbers
- FFB-Registry-01

Study Start
2014-06

Primary Completion (Estimated)
2037-06

Study Completion (Estimated)
2037-06

Enrollment (Estimated)
20000

Study Type
Observational [Patient Registry]

Study Contact
Name: Registry Coordinator
Phone Number: 800-683-5555 ext 1594
Email: Coordinator@MyRetinaTracker.org

United States
Maryland Locations

Columbia, Maryland, United States, 21045
Recruiting
Foundation Fighting Blindness

Contact
Registry Coordinator
800-683-5555 ext 1594 Coordinator@MyRetinaTracker.org
Principal Investigator:
Todd Durham, PhD

Eligibility Criteria
Description

Inclusion Criteria
- Diagnosed with an inherited retinal degenerative disease OR

Exclusion Criteria
- Glaucoma only
- Diabetic retinopathy only
- Non-retinal disease
- Not heritable retinal disease

Study Population
Affected individuals, all ages including minors registered by their parent or guardian.

Ages Eligible for Study
(Child, Adult, Older Adult)

Sexes Eligible for Study
All

Accepts Healthy Volunteers
Yes

Sampling Method
Probability Sample

Design Details
Observational Model: Other
Time Perspective: Prospective
Target Follow-up Duration: 20 Years

Primary outcome measures

Outcome measure	Measure description	Time frame
Number of participants with rare diagnoses within the inherited retinal degenerative disease category as defined by clinical evaluation	Participant profiles broken out to be disease category and genetic diagnosis	Data collection is ongoing, up to 20 years.

Sponsor
Foundation Fighting Blindness

Collaborators
No information provided

Investigators
• Principal Investigator: Todd Durham, PhD, Vice President, Clinical and Outcomes Research

General Publications
No publications available

United States

Recruiting

Stem Cell Ophthalmology Treatment Study II (SCOTS2)

ClinicalTrials.gov ID NCT03011541

Sponsor MD Stem Cells
Information provided by MD Stem Cells (Responsible Party)
Last Update Posted 2023-06-06

Study Overview

Brief Summary
This study will evaluate the use of autologous bone marrow-derived stem cells (BMSC) for the treatment of retinal and optic nerve damage or disease.

Detailed Description
Eyes with loss of vision from retinal or optic nerve conditions generally considered irreversible will be treated with a combination of injections of autologous bone marrow-derived stem cells isolated from the bone marrow using standard medical and surgical practices. Retinal conditions may include degenerative, ischemic, or physical damage (examples may include macular degeneration, hereditary retinal dystrophies such as retinitis pigmentosa, Stargardt, non-perfusion retinopathies, post-retinal detachment). Optic Nerve conditions may include degenerative, ischemic, or physical damage (examples may include optic nerve damage from glaucoma, compression, ischemic optic neuropathy, optic atrophy). Injections may include retrobulbar, subtenon, intravitreal, intraocular, subretinal, and intravenous. Patients will be followed for 12 months with serial comprehensive eye examinations including relevant imaging and diagnostic ophthalmic testing.

Official Title
Bone Marrow-Derived Stem Cell Ophthalmology Treatment Study II

Conditions
Retinal Disease
Age-Related Macular Degeneration
Retinitis Pigmentosa
Stargardt Disease
Optic Neuropathy
Nonarteritic Ischemic Optic Neuropathy
Optic Atrophy
Optic Nerve Disease
Glaucoma
Leber Hereditary Optic Neuropathy
Blindness
Vision Loss Night
Vision Loss Partial
Vision, Low
Retinopathy
Maculopathy
Macular Degeneration
Retina Atrophy

Intervention/Treatment
- Procedure: Arm 1

Other Study ID Numbers
- SCOTS2

Study Start (Actual)
2016-01

Primary Completion (Estimated)
2024-07

Study Completion (Estimated)
2025-07

Enrollment (Estimated)
500

Study Type
Interventional

Phase
Not Applicable

Study Contact
Name: Steven Levy, MD
Phone Number: 203-423-9494
Email: stevenlevy@mdstemcells.com

Study Contact Backup
Name: Steven Levy, MD
Phone Number: 203-423-9494
United States
Connecticut Locations

Westport, Connecticut, United States, 06880
Recruiting
MD Stem Cells

Contact
Steven Levy, MD
203-423-9494 stevenlevy@mdstemcells.com
Contact:
Steven Levy, MD
203-423-9494
Sub-Investigator:
Steven Levy, MD

Florida Locations

Coral Springs, Florida, United States, 33065
Recruiting
MD Stem Cells

Contact
Steven Levy, MD
203-423-9494

United Arab Emirates

Dubai, United Arab Emirates
Recruiting
Medcare Orthopaedics & Spine Hospital

Contact
Steven Levy, MD
(001) 2034239494

Eligibility Criteria
Description

Inclusion Criteria
- Have objective, documented damage to the retina or optic nerve unlikely to improve OR
- Have objective, documented damage to the retina or optic nerve that is progressive AND have less than or equal to 20/30 best-corrected central visual acuity in one or both eyes AND/OR an abnormal visual field in one or both eyes.

- Be at least 3 months postsurgical treatment intended to treat any ophthalmologic disease and stable.
- If under current medical therapy (pharmacologic treatment) for a retinal or optic nerve disease, be considered stable on that treatment, and unlikely to have visual function improvement (for example, glaucoma with intraocular pressure stable on topical medications but visual field damage).
- Have the potential for improvement with BMSC treatment and be at minimal risk of any potential harm from the procedure.
- Be over the age of 18
- Be medically stable and able to be medically cleared by their primary care physician or a licensed primary care practitioner for the procedure.
- Medical clearance means that in the estimation of the primary care practitioner, the patient can reasonably be expected to undergo the procedure without significant medical risk to health.

Exclusion Criteria
- Patients who are not capable of an adequate ophthalmologic examination or evaluation to document the pathology.
- Patients who are not capable or not willing to undergo follow-up eye exams with the principal investigator or their ophthalmologist or optometrist as outlined in the protocol.
- Patients who are not capable of providing informed consent.
- Patients who may be at significant risk to general health or to the eyes and visual function should they undergo the procedure.

Ages Eligible for Study
18 Years and older (Adult, Older Adult)

Sexes Eligible for Study
All

Accepts Healthy Volunteers
No

Design Details
Primary Purpose: Treatment
Allocation: N/A
Interventional Model: Single Group Assignment
Interventional Model Description: Single Arm- Arm 1. Comparator is natural history of the disease.
Masking: None (Open Label)

Arms and interventions

Participant group/arm	Intervention/treatment

Other: Arm 1
BMSC provided retrobulbar, subtenon, and intravenous for one or both eyes
	Procedure: Arm 1
	• Procedure/Surgery: RB (Retrobulbar)
	Retrobulbar injection of Bone Marrow-Derived Stem Cells (BMSC)
	Procedure/Surgery: ST (Subtenon)
	Subtenon injection of Bone Marrow-Derived Stem Cells (BMSC)
	Procedure/Surgery: IV (Intravenous)
	Intravenous injection of Bone Marrow-Derived Stem Cells (BMSC)
	• Other Names:
	  – Retrobulbar (RB)
	  – Subtenon (ST)
	  – Intravenous (IV)

Primary outcome measures

Outcome measure	Measure description	Time frame
Visual Acuity	Best-corrected visual acuity will be measured with Snellen Eye Chart and the ETDRS (Early Treatment Diabetic Retinopathy Study) Eye Chart when available at each post-procedure visit. Intervals at minimum will be first post-procedure day, then 3 months, 6 months, and 12 months post-procedure day. Recommended visit 1 month post-procedure day.	Change from pre-procedure to 12 months

Secondary outcome measures

Outcome measure	Measure description	Time frame
Visual Fields	Visual fields will be evaluated with automated perimetry during post-procedure visits as needed and specifically at 6 months and 12 months. Visual fields are a key measurement in patients with peripheral vision loss.	Change from pre-procedure to 12 months
Optical Coherence Tomography (OCT)	OCT thickness of the retinal nerve fiber layer, the optic nerve, and/or macula during the post-procedure visits as needed and specifically at 6 and 12 months – if available.	Change from pre-procedure to 12 months

Sponsor
MD Stem Cells

Collaborators
No information provided

Investigators
• Study Chair: Steven Levy, MD, MD Stem Cells
• Principal Investigator: Jeffrey Weiss, MD, Coral Springs

General Publications

- Weiss JN, Levy S. Stem Cell Ophthalmology Treatment Study (SCOTS): Bone Marrow-Derived Stem Cells in the Treatment of Stargardt Disease. Medicines 2021, 8(2), 10. https://doi.org/10.3390/medicines8020010

Abstract Background: Stargardt Disease is the most common inherited macular degeneration, typically resulting in progressive central vision loss and legal blindness at an early age. We report regarding 34 eyes with Stargardt Disease treated in the Stem Cell Ophthalmology Treatment Study (SCOTS and SCOTS2). Methods: Autologous bone marrow was processed, separating the stem cell fraction which was provided Arms using retrobulbar, subtenon, intravitreal or subretinal, and intravenous. The follow-up period was one year. Results: Of the 34 treated eyes, 21 (61.8%) improved, 8 (23.5%) remained stable, and 5 (14.7%) showed continued progression of their disease. Results were statistically significant with $p = 0.0004$. The average central vision improvement following treatment was 17.96% (95%CI, 16.39–19.53%) and ranged up to 80.5%. Of 17 patients treated, 13 (76.5%) showed visual acuity improvement in one or both eyes, 3 patients (17.6%) showed no net loss, and 1 worsened as a consequence of disease progression; 94.1% of patients had improved vision or remained stable. There were no adverse events. Conclusions: Patients with Stargardt Disease may potentially benefit from autologous bone marrow-derived stem cells (BMSC) as provided in SCOTS. Improvement or stabilization of vision was found to occur for the vast majority of reported patients and findings were highly statistically significant

Spain

Recruiting

Structural and Functional Characterization of Rare Ocular Diseases (RADIS)

ClinicalTrials.gov ID NCT05258032

Sponsor Barcelona Macula Foundation
Information provided by Marc Biarnes Perez, Barcelona Macula Foundation (Responsible Party)
Last Update Posted 2022-03-15

Study Overview

Brief Summary
Rare ocular diseases (ROD) are a heterogeneous group of ocular diseases that affect very few people and, generally, for which no treatment is available. An important

subgroup of these diseases are inherited retinal degenerations. In this study, we focus on understanding the natural history of different ROD that affect the posterior segment.

Official Title
Structural and Functional Characterization of Rare Ocular Diseases

Conditions
Retinitis Pigmentosa
Stargardt Disease
Best Disease
Pattern Dystrophy of Macula
Choroideremia

Intervention/Treatment

Other Study ID Numbers
• Barcelona Macula F

Study Start (Actual)
2021-11-24

Primary Completion (Estimated)
2024-11-24

Study Completion (Estimated)
2025-11-24

Enrollment (Estimated)
50

Study Type
Observational

Study Contact
Name: Marc Biarnes, PhD
Phone Number: +34935950155
Email: mbiarnes@barcelonamaculafound.org
Spain

Barcelona, Spain, 08022
Recruiting
Institut de la Màcula

Contact
Marc Biarnes, PhD
+34935950155 mbiarnes@barcelonamaculafound.org

Eligibility Criteria
Description

Inclusion Criteria
- Male or female 18 years or older with a diagnosis of a ROD affecting the posterior segment
- Patients able to undergo all required ophthalmic exams
- Patients able and willing to sign an informed consent

Exclusion Criteria
- Patients with other concomitant posterior segment disorders
- Patients taking drugs known to affect the retina and/or optic nerve
- Patients who underwent an intraocular surgery (aside from phacoemulsification with intraocular lens implantation), corneal, or glaucoma surgery
- Patients who have participated in the past 12 months or who are currently participating in clinical trials for an ocular disease

Study Population
Patients with a ROD affecting the posterior segment of the eye

Ages Eligible for Study
18 Years and older (Adult, Older Adult)

Sexes Eligible for Study
All

Accepts Healthy Volunteers
No
Sampling Method
Non-Probability Sample

Observational Model: Case-Only
Time Perspective: Prospective

Primary outcome measures

Outcome measure	Measure description	Time frame
Change in best-corrected visual acuity	Change from baseline in BCVA	Year 2 as compared to baseline

Secondary outcome measures

Outcome measure	Measure description	Time frame
Change in mean macular sensitivity	Change from baseline in mean macular sensitivity on microperimetry	Year 2 as compared to baseline
Change in retinal thickness	Change from baseline in central subfield retinal thickness on OCT	Year 2 as compared to baseline

Sponsor
Barcelona Macula Foundation

Collaborators
No information provided

Investigators
• No information provided

General Publications
No publications available

Switzerland

Recruiting

Function and Imaging Assessments for G1961E-associated Stargardt Disease (FIRSTORBIT)

ClinicalTrials.gov ID NCT05674058

Sponsor Institute of Molecular and Clinical Ophthalmology Basel
Information provided by Institute of Molecular and Clinical Ophthalmology Basel
    (Responsible Party)
Last Update Posted 2023-01-06

Study Overview

Brief Summary
Some phenotypes of Stargardt disease are rather distinct. These include the 'bull's eye maculopathy' phenotype associated with the frequent ABCA4 G1961E variant. In anticipation of a treatment trial, this natural history study aims to compare functional and structural outcome measures systematically.

Official Title
Function and Imaging Assessments for G1961E-associated Stargardt Disease:
    Outcome Measure Ranking as Basis for Interventional Trials

Conditions
Stargardt Disease
Stargardt Disease 1
Fundus Flavimaculatus
Macular Degeneration, Stargardt
Macular Dystrophy With Flecks, Type 1

Intervention/Treatment
• Other: No intervention

Other Study ID Numbers
• FIRSTORBIT

Study Start (Actual)
2022-11-01

Primary Completion (Estimated)
2025-10-31

Study Completion (Estimated)
2025-10-31

Enrollment (Estimated)
40

Study Type
Observational

Study Contact
Name: Maximilian Pfau, MD
Phone Number: +41 79 525 92 47
Email: maximilian.pfau@usb.ch
Switzerland
Basel-Stadt Locations

Basel, Basel-Stadt, Switzerland, CH-4031
Recruiting
University Hospital Basel

Contact
Maximilian Pfau, MD
+41 79 525 92 47 Maximilian.Pfau@usb.ch
Contact:
Kristina Pfau, MD
+41 79 357 36 93 Kristina.Pfau@usb.ch

Eligibility Criteria
Description

Inclusion Criteria
- Adult patients with G1961E-associated Stargardt disease
- Defined by (1) the presence of two pathogenic ABCA4 variants with at least one ABCA4G1961E variant, (2) a Stargardt disease phenotype, and (3) the absence of pathogenic variants in PRPH2, PROM1, and ELOVL4

Exclusion Criteria
- Inability to give informed consent
- Prior surgery (other than anti-VEGF injections, cataract surgery, YAG laser capsulotomy, or laser retinopexy) that – according to the investigator's judgment – may affect visual function assessments (e.g., retinal detachment surgery, glaucoma filtration surgery, or a history of a corneal transplant in the study-eye)

- Concurrent ophthalmic conditions in the study eye that (according to the investigator's judgment) may contribute to loss of vision such as clinically significant opacification of the ocular media (corneal dystrophies, cataract), other retinal diseases, or disease of the optic nerve head and visual pathway (including amblyopia)
- Major surgery planned or preclude study participation (according to the investigator's judgment)

Study Population

The study will include subjects with G1961E-associated Stargardt disease.

Ages Eligible for Study

18 Years and older (Adult, Older Adult)

Sexes Eligible for Study

All

Accepts Healthy Volunteers

No
Sampling Method
Non-Probability Sample

Study Plan

Design Details

Observational Model: Cohort
Time Perspective: Prospective

Cohorts and interventions

Intervention/treatment
Other: No intervention
• According to clinical practice.

Primary outcome measures

Outcome measure	Measure description	Time frame
Progression of photoreceptor outer and inner segment loss	Rate of change for the (square-root-transformed) EZ loss area (in mm/yr)	Two years from Baseline

Sponsor

Institute of Molecular and Clinical Ophthalmology Basel

Collaborators

No information provided

Investigators

No information provided

General Publications

- Pfau M, Cukras CA, Huryn LA, Zein WM, Ullah E, Boyle MP, Turriff A, Chen MA, Hinduja AS, Siebel HE, Hufnagel RB, Jeffrey BG, Brooks BP. Photoreceptor degeneration in ABCA4-associated retinopathy and its genetic correlates. JCI Insight. 2022 Jan 25;7(2):e155373. https://doi.org/10.1172/jci.insight.155373.
- Pfau M, Holz FG, Muller PL. Retinal light sensitivity as outcome measure in recessive Stargardt disease. Br J Ophthalmol. 2021 Feb;105(2):258–264. https://doi.org/10.1136/bjophthalmol-2020-316201. Epub 2020 Apr 28.

Chapter 4
Enrolling by Invitation Studies

United States

Non-interventional Long Term Follow-up Study of Participants Previously Enrolled in the STARLIGHT Study (SUSTAIN)

ClinicalTrials.gov ID NCT06048185

Sponsor Nanoscope Therapeutics Inc.
Information provided by Nanoscope Therapeutics Inc. (Responsible Party)
Last Update Posted 2023-10-13

Study Overview

Brief Summary
The current study is a non-interventional long-term safety follow-up of the subjects who completed STARLIGHT, in accordance with FDA guidance on recipients of human gene therapy products.

Detailed Description
This study is designed to follow subjects with Stargardt Disease (SD) previously enrolled in study NTXMCO-004 (STARLIGHT, NCT05417126). In that study, all 6 enrolled subjects received MCO-010, an ambient light-activated, Multi-Characteristic Opsin (MCO) transgene in an adeno-associated virus serotype 2 (AAV2) vector via intravitreal injection (IVT). MCO-010 has the potential to restore vision irrespective of the underlying gene mutation, and because it is directed at bipolar retinal cells, intact photoreceptors are not required. Further details on MCO-010 and the underlying disease under investigation are included in the protocol for STARLIGHT and are not repeated herein.

© The Author(s), under exclusive license to Springer Nature Switzerland AG 2024
J. N. Weiss, *Clinical Trials in Stargardt Disease Treatment*,
https://doi.org/10.1007/978-3-031-58807-5_4

Official Title
Long-Term Follow-up for Participants Who Previously Received a Single Intravitreal
Injection of MCO-010 Optogenetic Therapy in the STARLIGHT Study

Conditions
Stargardt Disease

Intervention/Treatment
• Biological: Gene Therapy Product-MCO-010

Other Study ID Numbers
• NTXLTFU-007

Study Start (Estimated)
2023-10

Primary Completion (Estimated)
2027-05

Study Completion (Estimated)
2027-07

Enrollment (Estimated)
6

Study Type
Observational

United States
Florida Locations

Miami, Florida, United States, 33136
Nanoscope Clinical Site

Texas Locations
McAllen, Texas, United States, 78503
Nanoscope Clinical Site

Eligibility Criteria
Description

Inclusion Criteria
Subjects are eligible to be included in the study only if all of the following criteria apply:

• Previously enrolled in study NTXMCO-004 study
• Able to comprehend and give informed consent.
• Able to comply with testing and all protocol tests.
• Agree to participate for the full 4-year study duration to the best of their abili-
ties and barring any unforeseen circumstances.

Exclusion Criteria

Not applicable. Subjects will be included in this study and will be consented after completion of all assessments at the Week 48 visit for the STARLIGHT study

Study Population

The study population eligible to participate will comprise of the 6 subjects previously enrolled in STARLIGHT.

Ages Eligible for Study

16 Years and older (Child, Adult, Older Adult)

Sexes Eligible for Study

All

Accepts Healthy Volunteers

No
Sampling Method
Non-Probability Sample

Design Details

Observational Model: Cohort
Time Perspective: Prospective
Biospecimen Retention: Samples With DNA
Biospecimen Description: Blood

Cohorts and interventions

Intervention/treatment
Biological: Gene Therapy Product-MCO-010 • The MCO-010 is an adeno-associated virus serotype 2-based vector that carried multi-characteristic opsin (MCO) gene expression cassette

Primary outcome measures

Outcome measure	Measure description	Time frame
Assessment of the long-term safety profile of a single intravitreal injection of MCO-010	Assessment of incidences, nature, and severity of treatment emergent adverse events (TEAEs), serious adverse events (SAEs), intraocular inflammation graded through ocular exam, clinical examination, and intraocular pressure.	204 weeks

Secondary outcome measures

Outcome measure	Measure description	Time frame
Evaluation of the long-term effects on visual acuity of a single intravitreal injection of MCO-010; 1.2E11 gc/eye	Change from baseline in BCVA over time in the study eye and fellow eye	204 weeks

Outcome measure	Measure description	Time frame
Exploration of the long-term impact of MCO-010 on retinal anatomy	Assessment of fundus photography and optical coherence tomography (OCT) outcomes over time	204 weeks
Assessment of the long-term durability of MCO-010 induced on gene reporter expression	Change from baseline of fundus fluorescence intensity of reporter (mCherry) over time in the study eye and fellow eye	204 weeks

Sponsor
Nanoscope Therapeutics Inc.

Collaborators
No information provided

Investigators
• Study Director: Dr. Samarendra Mohanty, Nanoscope Therapeutics Inc.

General Publications
No publications available

United States

Enrolling by Invitation

Open-Label Extension: Tolerability and Effects of ALK-001 on Stargardt Disease (TEASE)

ClinicalTrials.gov ID NCT04239625

Sponsor Alkeus Pharmaceuticals, Inc.
Information provided by Alkeus Pharmaceuticals, Inc. (Responsible Party)
Last Update Posted 2021-07-21

Study Overview

Brief Summary
The purpose of this open-label, multicenter study is to determine the long-term safety, pharmacokinetics, and effects of ALK-001 (C20-D3-retinyl acetate) on the progression of Stargardt disease. This study is an extension of NCT02402660 and enrolls participants who are at least 8 years old. Enrollment is by invitation only.

Funding Source – FDA OOPD

Official Title
A Phase 2 Multicenter, Double-Masked, Randomized, Placebo-Controlled Study to Investigate the Long Term Safety, Tolerability, Pharmacokinetics, and Effects of ALK-001 on the Progression of Stargardt Disease

Conditions

Stargardt Disease
Stargardt Macular Degeneration
Stargardt Macular Dystrophy
Autosomal Recessive Stargardt Disease 1 (ABCA4-related)

Intervention/Treatment

- Drug: ALK-001

Other Study ID Numbers

- ALK001-P1002-EXT
- R01FD004098 (U.S. FDA Grant/Contract)
- R01FD006016 (Other Grant/Funding Number) (OTHER_GRANT: FDA OOPD)

Study Start (Actual)

2019-12-20

Primary Completion (Estimated)

2024-12

Study Completion (Estimated)

2024-12

Enrollment (Estimated)

140

Study Type

Interventional

Phase

Phase 2

United States
Massachusetts Locations

Somerville, Massachusetts, United States, 02144
Coordinating Center

Eligibility Criteria
Description

Simplified Inclusion Criteria

- Clinical diagnosis of Stargardt disease (STGD1)
- Has at least two ABCA4 disease-causing mutations, unless authorized by sponsor
- Has a best-corrected visual acuity (BCVA) greater than approximately 20/160 in at least one eye
- Healthy as judged by investigator
- Able and willing to comply with study requirements, restrictions, and instructions and is likely to complete the 24-month study
- Has been invited to participate in this extension and has signed and dated the informed consent forms (or assent where appropriate) to participate
- Female of childbearing potential has signed the attestation on contraception requirements

Simplified Exclusion Criteria
- Is lactating or pregnant
- Has a medical condition likely to prevent compliance with the protocol and/or interfere with absorption of ALK-001 or performance of study procedures
- Has abnormal laboratory result(s) at screening
- Has an ocular disorder that may confound ocular assessments
- Has a history of ocular intervention within 90 days of screening

Ages Eligible for Study
8–70 Years (Child, Adult, Older Adult)

Sexes Eligible for Study
All

Accepts Healthy Volunteers
No

Design Details
Primary Purpose: Treatment
Allocation: N/A
Interventional Model: Single Group Assignment
Masking: None (Open Label)

Arms and interventions

Participant group/arm	Intervention/treatment

Experimental: ALK-001	Drug: ALK-001
	• Oral administration of a pill for up to 24 months
	• Other Names:
	  – C20-D3-Retinyl Acetate
	  – C20 Deuterated vitamin A

Primary outcome measures

Outcome measure	Measure description	Time frame
Safety and tolerability of ALK-001 assessed by incidence and/or clinically significant changes of a combination of ocular and non-ocular adverse events		From baseline to 24 months
Pharmacokinetic profile of ALK-001 derived from the concentrations of ALK-001 and metabolites in plasma		Up to 24 months

Sponsor
Alkeus Pharmaceuticals, Inc.

Collaborators
No information provided

Investigators
- Study Director: Leonide Saad, PhD, Alkeus Pharmaceuticals, Inc.

General Publications
- Ma L, Kaufman Y, Zhang J, Washington I. C20-D3-vitamin A slows lipofuscin accumulation and electrophysiological retinal degeneration in a mouse model of Stargardt disease. J Biol Chem. 2011 Mar 11;286(10):7966–7974. https://doi.org/10.1074/jbc.M110.178657. Epub 2010 Dec 14.
- Kaufman Y, Ma L, Washington I. Deuterium enrichment of vitamin A at the C20 position slows the formation of detrimental vitamin A dimers in wild-type rodents. J Biol Chem. 2011 Mar 11;286(10):7958–7965. https://doi.org/10.1074/jbc.M110.178640. Epub 2010 Nov 12.
- Mihai DM, Jiang H, Blaner WS, Romanov A, Washington I. The retina rapidly incorporates ingested C20-D(3)-vitamin A in a swine model. Mol Vis. 2013 Jul 25;19:1677–83. Print 2013.
- Charbel Issa P, Barnard AR, Herrmann P, Washington I, MacLaren RE. Rescue of the Stargardt phenotype in Abca4 knockout mice through inhibition of vitamin A dimerization. Proc Natl Acad Sci U S A. 2015 Jul 7;112(27):8415–20. https://doi.org/10.1073/pnas.1506960112. Epub 2015 Jun 23.
- Saad L, Washington I. Can Vitamin A be Improved to Prevent Blindness due to Age-Related Macular Degeneration, Stargardt Disease and Other Retinal Dystrophies? Adv Exp Med Biol. 2016;854:355–61. https://doi.org/10.1007/978-3-319-17121-0_47.

Chapter 5
Active, Not Recruiting Studies

United States

Phase I/II Follow-up Study of SAR422459 in Patients with Stargardt's Macular Degeneration

ClinicalTrials.gov ID NCT01736592

Sponsor Sanofi
Information provided by Sanofi (Responsible Party)
Last Update Posted 2023-06-02

Brief Summary
Primary Objective
To evaluate the long-term safety and tolerability of SAR422459 in patients with
　Stargardt's Macular Degeneration.
Secondary Objective:
To assess:

- Safety
- Biological activity

Detailed Description
Patients will be followed for 15 years after completion/early termination of the previous TDU13583 study (NCT01367444).

As the initial TDU13583 study is terminated - recruitment to this LTS13588
study is over with 27 patients enrolled.

Official Title
An Open Label Study to Determine the Long-Term Safety, Tolerability, and Biological
　Activity of SAR422459 in Patients With Stargardt's Macular Degeneration

J. N. Weiss, *Clinical Trials in Stargardt Disease Treatment*,
https://doi.org/10.1007/978-3-031-58807-5_5

Conditions
Stargardt's Disease

Intervention/Treatment
- Drug: Long-term follow-up in all patients who received SAR422459 in previous study TDU13583

Other Study ID Numbers
- LTS13588
- SG1/002/11

Study Start (Actual)
2012-12-14

Primary Completion (Estimated)
2033-08-29

Study Completion (Estimated)
2033-08-29

Enrollment (Actual)
27

Study Type
Interventional

Phase
Phase 1 and Phase 2

United States
Oregon Locations

Portland, Oregon, United States, 97239-3098
Investigational Site Number 840001

France

Paris, France, 75012
Investigational Site Number 250001

Eligibility Criteria
Description

Inclusion Criteria
Patients must meet ALL of the following criteria:

- Provide signed and dated written informed consent and any locally required authorization (e.g., Health Insurance Portability and Accountability Act [HIPAA])
- Must have been enrolled in protocol TDU13583 (SG1/001/10)
- Must have received a subretinal injection of SAR422459
- Must have completed protocol TDU13583 to Week 48 or undergone an early discontinuation visit.

Exclusion Criteria

The following would exclude patients from participation in the study:

- Did not receive SAR422459 as part of the TDU13583 protocol.

Ages Eligible for Study

6 Years and older (Child, Adult, Older Adult)

Sexes Eligible for Study

All

Accepts Healthy Volunteers

No

Design Details

Primary Purpose: Other
Allocation: N/A
Interventional Model: Single Group Assignment
Masking: None (Open Label)

Arms and interventions

Participant group/arm	Intervention/treatment
Other: Long-Term Follow-up Long-term follow-up in all patients who received SAR422459 in previous study TDU13583	Drug: Long-term follow-up in all patients who received SAR422459 in previous study TDU13583 • Blood draw for the laboratory assessment

Primary outcome measures

Outcome measure	Measure description	Time frame
The incidence of adverse events	The number and percentage of patients with treatment-emergent adverse events	15 years

Secondary outcome measures

Outcome measure	Measure description	Time frame
Clinically important changes in ocular safety assessments	From baseline in (TDU13583) study and from the last visit best-corrected visual acuity (BCVA), slit-lamp examination, fundoscopy, intraocular pressure, laboratory parameters, concomitant medications	baseline to 15 years
Delay in retinal degeneration	Measured as change from baseline in function relative to untreated contralateral eye on: BCVA, static perimetry, microperimetry, autofluorescence, optical coherence tomography (OCT)	baseline to 15 years

Sponsor
Sanofi

Collaborators
No information provided

Investigators
- Principal Investigator: David Wilson, MD, Oregon Health and Science University
- Principal Investigator: José-Alain Sahel, MD, Centre National d'Ophtalmologie des Quinze-Vingts

General Publications
No publications available

United States

Active, Not Recruiting

Safety and Effects of a Single Intravitreal Injection of vMCO-010 Optogenetic Therapy in Subjects with Stargardt Disease (STARLIGHT)

ClinicalTrials.gov ID NCT05417126

Sponsor Nanoscope Therapeutics Inc.
Information provided by Nanoscope Therapeutics Inc. (Responsible Party)
Last Update Posted 2023-10-23

Brief Summary
The purpose of the study is to evaluate the safety and effects of a single intravitreal injection of virally carried Multi-Characteristic Opsin (vMCO-010) in Subjects with Stargardt Disease

Detailed Description
This multicenter open label study will evaluate single dose level of vMCO-010 in up to 6 subjects with Stargardt's Disease. Subjects with documented clinical diagnosis of Stargardt disease (classic fleck phenotype and/or well-demarcated subfoveal area of significantly reduced autofluorescence as imaged by FAF), or genetic diagnosis with pathogenic variants in ABCA4, ELOVL4, or PROM 1. All subjects will continue to be assessed for 48 weeks following treatment with vMCO-010.

Official Title
A Phase 2a, Open Label Multicenter Clinical Trial to Evaluate the Safety and Effects of a Single Intravitreal Injection of vMCO-010 Optogenetic Therapy in Subjects With Stargardt Disease

Conditions
Stargardt Disease

Intervention/Treatment
- Biological: Gene Therapy-vMCO-010

Other Study ID Numbers
- NTXMCO-004

Study Start (Actual)
2022-07-05

Primary Completion (Actual)
2023-09-28

Study Completion (Estimated)
2023-10

Enrollment (Actual)
6

Study Type
Interventional

Phase
Phase 2

United States
Florida Locations

Miami, Florida, United States, 33136
Nanoscope Clinical Site

Texas Locations

McAllen, Texas, United States, 78503
Nanoscope Clinical Site

Eligibility Criteria
Description

Inclusion Criteria
- ≥ 16 years of age
- Able to comprehend and give informed consent.
- Able to comply with testing and all protocol tests.
- Documented clinical diagnosis of Stargardt disease (classic fleck phenotype and/ or well-demarcated sub-foveal area of significantly reduced autofluorescence as imaged by FAF), or genetic diagnosis with pathogenic variants in ABCA4, ELOVL4, or PROM1

- In the study eye: ETDRS BCVA in range of 1.3 logMAR (Approximate Snellen equivalent: 20/400) to 1.9 logMAR (Snellen equivalent: 20/1600), and ETDRS BCVA no better than 20/200 in the fellow eye.
- Presence of retinal inner nuclear and nerve fiber layers on optical coherence tomography (OCT) testing in the study eye at screening

Exclusion Criteria
- Presence of any concurrent ocular disease that would affect study outcomes (e.g., severe cataracts; subjects can be enrolled 3 months after successful cataract surgery).
- Received any of the following treatments: gene therapy, stem cell therapy, surgical implantation of prosthetic retinal chips (such as ARGUS-II), or subretinal injections.
- Has taken non-approved items (supplement containing vitamin A or beta-carotene, liver-based products, or prescription oral retinoid medications) over the past 30 days
- Participation in an interventional study of a vitamin A derivative $\leq$ 3 months prior to screening
- Presence of significant cardiovascular or cerebrovascular disease, including stroke within 12 months of entry.
- Resting heart rate outside specified limits upon repeated measurement.
- History of uncontrolled diabetes, hepatitis, pancreatitis, cirrhosis, liver failure, uncontrolled thyroid disease, or hypervitaminosis A.
- Any intraocular surgery or thermal laser within 3 months of trial entry or any prior thermal laser in the macular region.
- Any major surgical procedure within one month of trial entry or anticipated during the trial.
- Clinically significant abnormal lab results at screening
- Known serious allergies to the fluorescein dye used in angiography or intraocular pressure measurement, povidone iodine, or to the components of the vMCO-010 formulation
- In the Investigator's opinion, any severe acute or chronic medical condition, psychiatric condition, physical examination finding, or laboratory abnormality
- Preexisting conditions in the study eye such as glaucoma, diseases affecting the optic nerve causing significant visual field loss, history of uveitis, corneal, or lenticular opacities.
- Presence of any complicating systemic diseases such as malignancies whose treatment could affect central nervous system function.
- Subjects who are positive for syphilis, hepatitis B, C, and human immunodeficiency virus (HIV) will be excluded.
- Presence of narrow iridocorneal angles contraindicating pupillary dilation in the study eye.

- Presence of disorders of the ocular media in the study eye which could interfere with visual acuity and other ocular assessments, including OCT, during the study period.
- Presence of macular hole in the study eye, evident by ophthalmoscopy and/or by OCT examinations
- Current evidence of retinal detachment in the study eye assessed by the investigator that significantly affects central vision.
- Current use of hydroxychloroquine, chloroquine, or any related retina-toxic compounds.
- Active ocular inflammation or recurrent history of idiopathic or autoimmune-associated uveitis.

Ages Eligible for Study
16 Years and older (Child, Adult, Older Adult)

Sexes Eligible for Study
All

Accepts Healthy Volunteers
No

Design Details
Primary Purpose: Treatment
Allocation: N/A
Interventional Model: Single Group Assignment
Interventional Model Description: 6 subjects will be enrolled for vMCO-010 treatment
Masking: None (Open Label)

Arms and interventions

Participant group/arm	Intervention/treatment
Experimental: Experimental-vMCO-010 Participants receive 1.2E11gc/eye of vMCO-010	Biological: Gene Therapy-vMCO-010 • The vMCO-010 is an adeno-associated virus serotype 2-based vector-carried multi-characteristic opsin (MCO) gene expression cassette

Primary outcome measures

Outcome measure	Measure description	Time frame
Type, severity, and incidence of ocular and systemic adverse events (AEs)	Type, severity, and incidence of ocular and systemic adverse events (AEs), specifically those related to intravitreal injection of vMCO-010	48 weeks

Secondary outcome measures

Outcome measure	Measure description	Time frame
Effect of vMCO-010 as assessed by visual acuity	Change from baseline in BCVA at Weeks 12, 24, and 48 in the study eye and the fellow eye	48 weeks
Effect of vMCO-010 on Light-guided Mobility	Change from baseline in Multi-Luminance Mobility Test at weeks 12, 24, and 48 in the study eye and the fellow eye	48 Weeks
Effect of vMCO-010 on determination of shape	Change from baseline in accuracy in determination of shape using Low Vision Multiparameter Test (LVMPT) at weeks 12, 24, and 48 in the study eye and the fellow eye	48 Weeks
Effect of vMCO-010 on determination of optical flow	Change from baseline in accuracy in determination of optical flow using the LVMPT at weeks 12, 24, and 48 in the study eye and the fellow eye	48 Weeks

Sponsor
Nanoscope Therapeutics Inc.

Collaborators
No information provided

Investigators
- Study Director: Dr Samarendra Mohanty, Nanoscope Therapeutics Inc.

General Publications
No publications available

United States

Active, Not Recruiting

Study to Evaluate the Safety and Efficacy of Tinlarebant in the Treatment of Stargardt Disease in Adolescent Subjects Lesion(s) in Adolescent Subjects with STGD1 (DRAGON)

ClinicalTrials.gov ID NCT05244304

Sponsor Belite Bio, Inc
Information provided by Belite Bio, Inc (Responsible Party)
Last Update Posted 2023-08-01

Brief Summary
The primary objective of this trial is to assess the efficacy of Tinlarebant in slowing the rate of growth of atrophic lesion(s) in adolescent subjects with STGD1

Detailed Description

Approximately 90 subjects will be enrolled in this study. Subjects will be assigned to study drug (Tinlarebant 5 mg/placebo) with treatment period of up to 24 months with 28 days of follow-up.

Official Title

Phase 3, Multicenter, Randomized, Double-Masked, Placebo-Controlled Study to Evaluate the Safety and Efficacy of Tinlarebant in the Treatment of Stargardt Disease in Adolescent Subjects

Conditions

Stargardt Disease 1

Intervention/Treatment

- Drug: Tinlarebant
- Drug: Placebo

Other Study ID Numbers

- LBS-008-CT03

Study Start (Actual)

2022-03-28

Primary Completion (Estimated)

2025-08

Study Completion (Estimated)

2025-10

Enrollment (Actual)

90

Study Type

Interventional

Phase

Phase 3

United States
California Locations

Palo Alto, California, United States, 94303
Belite Study Site

Florida Locations

Gainesville, Florida, United States, 32607
Belite Study Site

Minnesota Locations

Minneapolis, Minnesota, United States, 55435
Belite Study Site

New York Locations

New York, New York, United States, 10032
Belite Study Site

Utah Locations

Salt Lake City, Utah, United States, 84132
Belite Study Site

Australia

South Brisbane, Australia
Belite Study Site

New South Wales Locations

Westmead, New South Wales, Australia
Belite Study Site

Victoria Locations

East Melbourne, Victoria, Australia
Belite Study Site

Belgium

Gent, Belgium
Belite Study Site

Leuven, Belgium
Belite Study Site

China

Beijing, China
Belite Study Site

Shanghai, China
Belite Study Site

France

Paris, France
Belite Study Site

Germany

Bonn, Germany
Belite Study Site

Gießen, Germany
Belite Study Site

Tübingen, Germany
Belite Study Site

Hong Kong

Kowloon, Hong Kong
Belite Study Site

Netherlands

Amsterdam, Netherlands
Belite Study Site

Nijmegen, Netherlands
Belite Study Site

Switzerland

Basel, Switzerland
Belite Study Site

Taiwan

Taipei, Taiwan
Belite Study Site

Taoyuan City, Taiwan
Belite Study Site

United Kingdom

London, United Kingdom
Belite Study Site

Southampton, United Kingdom
Belite Study Site

Eligibility Criteria
Description

Inclusion Criteria
- Male or female subjects 12–20 years old, inclusive.
- Subject must have clinically diagnosed STGD1 (Stargardt disease 1) with at least 1 mutation identified in the ABCA4 gene.
- Subject must have a defined aggregate atrophic lesion size within 3 disc areas (7.62 mm^2), as imaged by FAF in the study eye. Subjects must have a BCVA of 20/200 or better for the study eye based on ETDRS letter score
- Subject and their parent(s) or legal guardian are willing to provide their consent on an Institutional Review Board (IRB)/Independent Ethics Committee (IEC)/ Human Research Ethics Committee (HREC)-approved informed consent form (ICF) prior to participating in any study-related procedures.
- Subject agrees to comply with all protocol requirements.

Exclusion Criteria

- Any ocular disease other than Stargardt (STGD1) at baseline that, in the opinion of the investigator, would complicate assessment of a treatment effect.
- History of ocular surgery in the study eye in the last 3 months.
- Investigational drug use of any kind in the last 3 months or within 5 half-lives of the investigational drug, whichever is shorter.
- Any prior gene therapy.
- Vitamin A (retinol) deficiency as defined as a retinol serum level less than 20 mcg/dL (=0.7 µmol/L).

Ages Eligible for Study
12–20 Years (Child, Adult)

Sexes Eligible for Study
All

Accepts Healthy Volunteers
No

Design Details
Primary Purpose: Treatment
Allocation: Randomized
Interventional Model: Parallel Assignment
Interventional Model Description: This is a Phase 3 randomized, double-masked, parallel group, multicenter study to evaluate the efficacy and safety of Tinlarebant 5 mg in the treatment of adolescent subjects with STGD1.
Masking: Double (Participant Investigator)
Masking Description: Eligible subjects will be randomly assigned to begin treatment in 2:1 ratio to receive the study drug (either Tinlarebant 5 mg or matching placebo)

Arms and interventions

Participant group/arm	Intervention/treatment
Experimental: Tinlarebant 5 mg tablet taken orally once a day	Drug: Tinlarebant • Tinlarebant drug substance is a white to off-white substance and is dispensed as a tablet for oral administration.
Placebo Comparator: Placebo Placebo tablets for Tinlarebant 5 mg are prepared similarly but use microcrystalline cellulose, NF, in place of the active drug substance and will be identical in size and appearance.	Drug: Placebo • Not active drug

Primary outcome measures

Outcome measure	Measure description	Time frame
To measure change in atrophic lesion size (definitely decreased autofluorescence, DDAF) by fundus autofluorescence (FAF) photography from baseline		Baseline through month 24

Secondary outcome measures

Outcome measure	Measure description	Time frame
To measure the change in retinal thickness assessed by spectral-domain optical coherence tomography (SD-OCT) from baseline		Baseline through month 24
To measure the change in retinal morphology assessed by spectral-domain optical coherence tomography (SD-OCT) from baseline		Baseline through month 24
To measure change in BCVA (Best-Corrected Visual Acuity) score measured by the EDTRS method from baseline		Baseline through month 24
To measure change in plasma concentration of RBP4 levels (μM) from baseline		Baseline through month 24
The correlation between change in plasma RBP4 level and the rate of lesion size growth (definitely decreased autofluorescence, DDAF) by fundus autofluorescence (FAF) photography from baseline		Baseline through month 24
To assess the systemic and ocular safety and tolerability of Tinlarebant	Frequency, duration, and severity of AEs	Baseline through month 24

Other outcome measures

Outcome measure	Measure description	Time frame
To measure change in total decreased autofluorescence (DAF) by FAF photography from baseline		Baseline through month 24
To measure change in questionably decreased autofluorescence (QDAF) by FAF photography from baseline		Baseline through month 24
To measure change in quantitative autofluorescence (qAF) level from baseline		Baseline through month 24
To measure change in retinal sensitivity by microperimetry from baseline		Baseline through month 24

Sponsor
Belite Bio, Inc

Collaborators
No information provided

Investigators
No information provided

General Publications
No publications available

United States

Active, Not Recruiting

Zimura Compared to Sham in Patients with Autosomal Recessive Stargardt Disease (STGD1)

ClinicalTrials.gov ID NCT03364153

Sponsor IVERIC bio, Inc.
Information provided by IVERIC bio, Inc. (Responsible Party)
Last Update Posted 2023-10-04

Study Overview

Brief Summary
To evaluate the safety and efficacy of Zimura™ (complement factor C5 inhibitor) compared to Sham in subjects with autosomal recessive Stargardt disease 1 (STGD1).

Official Title
A Phase 2b Randomized, Double-masked, Controlled Trial to Establish the Safety and Efficacy of Zimura™ (Complement C5 Inhibitor) Compared to Sham in Subjects With Autosomal Recessive Stargardt Disease

Conditions
Stargardt Disease 1

Intervention/Treatment
- Drug: Zimura
- Other: Sham

Other Study ID Numbers
- OPH2005

Study Start (Actual)
2018-01-12

Primary Completion (Estimated)
2025-04

Study Completion (Estimated)
2025-04

Enrollment (Estimated)
120

Study Type
Interventional

Phase
Phase 2

United States
Arizona Locations

Phoenix, Arizona, United States, 85053
Retinal Research Institute

California Locations

Los Angeles, California, United States, 90095
Jules Stein Eye Institute/David Geffen School of Medicine

Florida Locations

Gainesville, Florida, United States, 32607
VitreoRetinal Associates

Pensacola, Florida, United States, 32503
Retina Specialty Institute

Maryland Locations

Baltimore, Maryland, United States, 21287
Wilmer Eye Institute, Johns Hopkins

Massachusetts Locations

Boston, Massachusetts, United States, 02114
Ophthalmic Consultants of Boston

Michigan Locations

Ann Arbor, Michigan, United States, 48105
University of Michigan/Kellogg Eye Center

Minnesota Locations

Minneapolis, Minnesota, United States, 55404
The Retina Center

New Jersey Locations

Bloomfield, New Jersey, United States, 07003
Envision Ocular, LLC

Oregon Locations

Portland, Oregon, United States, 97239
Casey Eye Institute/Oregon Health & Science University

Pennsylvania Locations

Philadelphia, Pennsylvania, United States, 19107

Wills Eye Hospital/Mid Atlantic Retina

Pittsburgh, Pennsylvania, United States, 15213
UPMC Eye Center

South Carolina Locations

West Columbia, South Carolina, United States, 29169
Palmetto Retina Center

Texas Locations

Austin, Texas, United States, 78705
Austin Retina Associates

Bellaire, Texas, United States, 77401
Retina Consultants of Texas

Dallas, Texas, United States, 75231
Retina Foundation of the Southwest

Willow Park, Texas, United States, 76087
Strategic Clinical Research Group

Utah Locations

Salt Lake City, Utah, United States, 84132
University of Utah John A. Moran Eye Center

France

Créteil, France, 94010
Creteil University Eye Clinic University Paris EST

Paris, France, 75012
Centre ophtalmologique des Quinzes Vingts

Rhone-Alpes Locations

Lyon, Rhone-Alpes, France, 69004
Hopital de la Croix-Rousse

Germany

Bonn, Germany, 53127
University of Bonn

München, Germany, 80336
Augenklinik der LMU München

Tübingen, Germany, 72076
University of Tuebingen

Hungary

Budapest, Hungary, 1133

Budapest Retina Institute

Budapest, Hungary, H-1083
Semmelweis Egyetem

Debrecen, Hungary, 4032
University of Debrecen DE KK Szemészeti Klinika

Pécs, Hungary, 7621
Ganglion Medical Center

Szeged, Hungary, 6720
Szegedi Tudomanyegyetem, Szent-Gyorgyi Albert Klinikai Kozpont,
  Szemeszeti Klinika

Israel

Haifa, Israel, 3109601
Rambam Health Care Campus

Jerusalem, Israel, 9112001
Hadassah University Hospital

Petah tikva, Israel, 4941492
Rabin Medical Center, Beilinson campus

Rehovot, Israel, 7610001
Kaplan Medical Center

Tel Aviv, Israel, 6423906
Tel-Aviv Sourasky Medical Center, Ichilov Hospital

Italy

Bologna, Italy, 40138
AOU Policlinico Sant'Orsola Malpighi, U.O. Oftalmologia,

Florence, Italy, 50121
Azienda Ospedaliera Universitaria Careggi

Milano, Italy, 20132
Ospedale San Raffaele

Naples, Italy, 80131
University of Campania Luigi Vanvitelli Eye Clinic

Rome, Italy, 00133
Fondazione Policlinico Tor Vergata, UOSD Patologie Retiniche

Spain

Barcelona, Spain, 08022
Institut de la Macula

United Kingdom

Edinburgh, United Kingdom, EH3 9HA
Princess Alexandra Eye Pavillion

London, United Kingdom, EC1V 2PD
Moorfields Eye Hospital

Eligibility Criteria
Description

Inclusion Criteria
- At least two pathogenic mutations of ABCA4 gene confirmed by a CLIA-certified laboratory
- Best-corrected visual acuity in the study eye between 20/20 and 20/200 Snellen equivalent, inclusive

Exclusion Criteria
- Macular atrophy secondary to any condition other than STGD1 in either eye
- Any prior treatment for STGD1 including gene therapy, stem cell therapy, or any prior intravitreal treatment for any indication in either eye
- Participation in an interventional study of a vitamin A derivative $\leq$ 3 months prior to screening
- Presence of intraocular inflammation, macular hole, pathologic myopia, epiretinal membrane, evidence of significant vitreo-macular traction, vitreous hemorrhage, or aphakia
- Any intraocular surgery or thermal laser within 3 months of trial entry. Any prior thermal laser in the macular region
- Diabetes mellitus
- HbA1c value of $\geq 6.5\%$
- Stroke within 12 months of trial entry
- Any major surgical procedure within one month of trial entry or anticipated during the trial
- Any treatment with an investigational agent in the past 60 days for any condition
- Women who are pregnant or nursing
- Known serious allergies to the fluorescein dye used in angiography, povidone iodine, or to the components of the Zimura formulation

Ages Eligible for Study
18–60 Years (Adult)

Sexes Eligible for Study
All

Accepts Healthy Volunteers
No

Design Details
Primary Purpose: Treatment
Allocation: Randomized

Interventional Model: Parallel Assignment
Masking: Triple (Participant Investigator Outcomes Assessor)

Arms and interventions

Participant group/arm	Intervention/treatment
Experimental: Cohort 1 Zimura dose group	Drug: Zimura • Zimura Intravitreal Injection • Other Names: – avacincaptad pegol
Sham Comparator: Cohort 2 Sham dose group	Other: Sham • Sham Intravitreal Injection

Primary outcome measures

Outcome measure	Measure description	Time frame
Spectral-Domain Optical Coherence Tomography (SD-OCT)	Mean rate of change in the area of ellipsoid zone defect measured by en face SD-OCT	18 months

Sponsor
IVERIC bio, Inc.

Collaborators
No information provided

Investigators
No information provided

General Publications
No publications available

United States

Active, Not Recruiting

Natural History of Eye Diseases Related to ABCA4 Mutations

ClinicalTrials.gov ID NCT01736293

Sponsor National Eye Institute (NEI)
Information provided by National Institutes of Health Clinical Center (CC) (National Eye Institute (NEI)) (Responsible Party)
Last Update Posted 2023-10-27

Brief Summary
Background
- The ABCA4 gene contains a blueprint for the ABCA4 protein. When this protein is absent or faulty (such as in Stargardt's disease), waste material from dead cells collects in the eye. The waste material may cause other cells in the eye to die. This can lead to the loss of vision. Researchers want to look at blood and skin samples from people with ABCA4 gene mutations to study-related eye diseases.

Objectives
- To study eye diseases that are related to mutations in the ABCA4 gene.

Eligibility
- Individuals at least 12 years of age who have ABCA4 gene mutations.

Design
- The study requires 12 visits to the National Eye Institute clinic over 10 years. In the first year, there will be three visits. After the first year, participants will have one visit a year for 9 more years.
- Participants will be screened with a physical exam, full eye exam, and medical history. The eye exam will check eye pressure, light and color sensitivity, and retina function.
- Participants will provide a blood sample and a skin tissue sample for study.
- No treatment will be provided as part of this study.

Detailed Description
Objectives
The objectives of this study are to (1) establish a cohort of participants with ABCA4-related retinopathies in anticipation of future clinical trials, (2) create a repository of plasma, DNA, and skin fibroblast samples from the accrued cohort of ABCA4-related retinopathy participants, (3) formulate clinical outcome measures for future studies, and (4) acquire and perform preliminary analyses of data that may advance our understanding of genotype-phenotype correlations in ABCA4-related retinopathies.

In addition, the skin fibroblast samples collected from participants may be used to generate iPS cells, which may be differentiated into RPE and/or neural retinal cells. These cells, if produced, will be used to analyze molecular mechanisms involved in disease pathogenesis and to perform high-throughput (HTP) drug screens to identify novel potential therapeutic compounds.

Study Population
Sixty-five (65) participants, age 12 or above, with ABCA4-related retinopathies, will be initially accrued for this study. However, up to an additional five participants may be enrolled to replace participants who may withdraw from the study prior to reaching the Month 12 visit.

Design

In this natural history study, participants will be followed for 10 years. Because three years may be required to enroll 65 participants, this study will last up to 13 years. Participants will be recruited through other preexisting NIH protocols, such as the Ocular Natural History Protocol (16-EI-0134), The Genetics of Inherited Eye Disease Protocol (15-EI-0128), the NEI Screening Protocol (08-EI-0102), and the National Ophthalmic Disease Genotyping and Phenotyping Network, Phase II protocol (eyeGENE II, 10-EI-N164), or through referral from an outside clinician after a review of pertinent medical records and genetic testing. All participants will undergo a standardized medical/ophthalmic history and a complete baseline eye examination, which may include noninvasive electrophysiology (e.g., electroretinography), psychophysiology (e.g., microperimetry, static perimetry), and diagnostic imaging examinations (e.g., optical coherence tomography).

The participants will be examined three times over the course of the first year (i.e., baseline examination, Month 6, and Month 12). After the first year, they will return to the NEI clinic on an annual basis for the next nine years. This study will require a minimum of 12 study visits. Participants may be seen at more frequent intervals at the investigators' discretion, depending on the clinical and research situation. Participants will be required to submit a blood sample as part of the study for DNA and serum banking, and they will have the option to provide a 3-mm punch skin biopsy to facilitate research at a cellular level.

Outcome Measures

The primary outcome for this study is the establishment of a cohort of participants with ABCA4-related retinopathies, and the secondary outcome is the creation of a repository of plasma, DNA, and skin fibroblast samples from the accrued cohort of ABCA4-related retinopathy participants. Exploratory outcomes for this study include: (1) the formulation of clinical outcome measures for future studies and (2) the acquisition and preliminary analysis of data that may advance our understanding of genotype-phenotype correlations in ABCA4-related retinopathies. Potential exploratory outcomes include: (1) the generation of iPS cells from the skin fibroblast samples, (2) the differentiation of the generated iPS cells into RPE and/or neural retinal cells, and (3) the use of the participant-specific RPE and/or neural retinal cells to perform HTP drug screens to identify novel potential therapeutic compounds. The cells obtained in this protocol may be genetically modified and may be used for in vivo research.

Official Title

Natural History of ABCA4-Related Retinopathies

Conditions

Retinal Degeneration
ABCA4-Related Retinopathies

Intervention/Treatment

Other Study ID Numbers
- 120203
- 12-EI-0203

Study Start (Actual)
2012-10-09

Primary Completion
Study Completion

Enrollment (Actual)
68

Study Type
Observational

United States
Maryland Locations

Bethesda, Maryland, United States, 20892
National Institutes of Health Clinical Center

Eligibility Criteria
Description

Inclusion Criteria
- Participant must be 12 years of age or older.
- Participant (or legal guardian) must understand and sign the protocol's informed consent document.
- Participant must be able to cooperate with detailed psychophysics and electrophysiology testing.
- Participant must be able to provide a blood sample.
- Participant has:

  - A maculopathy or retinal degeneration plus two (or more) clear mutations in the ABCA4 gene (ascertained with CLIA-certified testing) that are known to be associated with retinal disease,

OR
One clear mutation in ABCA4 associated with a classic presentation of fundus flavimaculatus/Stargardt macular dystrophy (e.g., flecks, macular atrophy) and no pathogenic mutation(s) in other genes known to cause macular dystrophy.

OR
One clear mutation in ABCA4, a cone-rod degeneration, and no clearly pathogenic mutation(s) in other genes known to cause cone-rod degeneration.

Exclusion Criteria
Participant has evidence of a systemic condition or ocular disease not related to ABCA4 mutations that would complicate the analysis of psychophysical, electrophysiological, or imaging data. For example, a participant with advanced dia-

betes mellitus and significant diabetic retinopathy may display changes in retinal function that could be related to either his/her diabetic retinopathy or ABCA4 mutations.

Study Population

Participants will be recruited from other NEI protocols, such as the Ocular Natural History Protocol (16-EI-0134), the Genetics of Inherited Eye Disease Protocol (15-EI-0128), the NEI Screening Protocol (08-EI-0102), and/or the National Ophthalmic Disease Genotyping and Phenotyping Network, Phase II Protocol (eyeGENE II, 10-EI-N164), or through referral from an outside clinician after a review of pertinent medical records and genetic test results.

Ages Eligible for Study

12–100 Years (Child, Adult, Older Adult)

Sexes Eligible for Study

All

Accepts Healthy Volunteers

No
Sampling Method
Non-Probability Sample

Design Details

Observational Model: Cohort
Time Perspective: Prospective

Cohorts and interventions

Group/cohort
Affected Participants Participants with ABCA4-related retinopathies.

Primary outcome measures

Outcome measure	Measure description	Time frame
Establish cohort	Establish a cohort of participants with ABCA4 retinopathies in anticipation of future clinical trials.	Over the study duration

Sponsor

National Eye Institute (NEI)

Collaborators

No information provided

Investigators

- Principal Investigator: Brian P Brooks, M.D., National Eye Institute (NEI)

General Publications
- Allikmets R. A photoreceptor cell-specific ATP-binding transporter gene (ABCR) is mutated in recessive Stargardt macular dystrophy. Nat Genet. 1997 Sep;17(1):122. https://doi.org/10.1038/ng0997-122a. No abstract available.
- Gomes NL, Greenstein VC, Carlson JN, Tsang SH, Smith RT, Carr RE, Hood DC, Chang S. A comparison of fundus autofluorescence and retinal structure in patients with Stargardt disease. Invest Ophthalmol Vis Sci. 2009 Aug;50(8):3953–9. https://doi.org/10.1167/iovs.08-2657. Epub 2009 Mar 25.
- Gonzalez F, Boue S, Izpisua Belmonte JC. Methods for making induced pluripotent stem cells: reprogramming a la carte. Nat Rev Genet. 2011 Apr;12(4):231–42. https://doi.org/10.1038/nrg2937. Epub 2011 Feb 22.

Australia

Active, Not Recruiting

This is a Dose-finding Study Followed by 2-year Extension Study to Evaluate Safety and Tolerability of Tinlarebant in Adolescent Subjects with Stargardt Disease

ClinicalTrials.gov ID NCT05266014

Sponsor RBP4 Pty Ltd
Information provided by RBP4 Pty Ltd (Responsible Party)
Last Update Posted 2022-04-26

Study Overview

Brief Summary
Stargardt disease 1 (STGD1) is the most prevalent form of juvenile macular degeneration. It is caused by a rare, inherited autosomal recessive trait, leading to severe and irreversible blindness by the first or second decade of life. Earlier onset of the disease is related to a rapid vision loss, while patients with a later onset tend to have a better prognosis.

This study will enroll subjects aged 12–18 years old with a confirmed clinical diagnosis of Stargardt disease type 1 (STGD1). This study will include 2 phases, the phase 1b portion is to determine the optimal dose for phase 2 based on the extent of retinol-binding protein 4 (RBP4) reduction after 2 cycles of Tinlarebant treatment. The phase 2 portion will evaluate the safety and efficacy of a single daily dose of Tinlarebant over a 24-month treatment period.

Official Title
Phase 1/2, Open-Label, Dose-Finding Followed by 2-Year Extension Study to Evaluate Safety and Tolerability of Tinlarebant in Adolescent Subjects With Stargardt Disease

Conditions
Stargardt Disease

Intervention/Treatment
- Drug: Tinlarebant

Other Study ID Numbers
- LBS-008-CT02

Study Start (Actual)
2021-03-12

Primary Completion (Estimated)
2023-08-22

Study Completion (Estimated)
2023-08-22
Enrollment (Actual)
13

Study Type
Interventional

Phase
Phase 1 and Phase 2

Australia
New South Wales Locations

Westmead, New South Wales, Australia, 2145
Sydney Children's Hospitals Network

Western Australia Locations

Perth, Western Australia, Australia, 6009
Lions Eye Institute

Taiwan

Taipei, Taiwan, 100
National Taiwan University Hospital

Eligibility Criteria
Description

Major Inclusion Criteria
Subject must have clinically diagnosed Stargardt disease with at least one mutation
identified in the ABCA4 gene.

Major Exclusion Criteria
Any ocular disease other than Stargardt disease at baseline that, in the opinion of the
PI, would complicate assessment of a treatment effect.

Ages Eligible for Study
12–18 Years (Child, Adult)

Sexes Eligible for Study
All

Accepts Healthy Volunteers
No
Study Plan

Design Details
Primary Purpose: Treatment
Allocation: N/A
Interventional Model: Single Group Assignment
Masking: None (Open Label)

Arms and interventions

Participant group/arm	Intervention/treatment
Experimental: Tinlarebant Daily, oral administration of one Tinlarebant.	Drug: Tinlarebant • Phase 1b Portion: Tinlarebant will be self-administered orally once daily for 2 cycles, 14 days per cycle. • Phase 2 portion: Tinlarebant will be self-administered orally once daily for 24 months.

Primary outcome measures

Outcome measure	Measure description	Time frame
To evaluate systemic and ocular safety and tolerability of Tinlarebant.	To evaluate safety and tolerability of daily dosing of Tinlarebant assessed by incidence and/or severity of ocular and non-ocular adverse events.	From baseline to 24 months
The optimal dose for Phase 2.	To determine optimal dose of Tinlarebant administered orally in adolescent patients with Stargardt Disease.	Up to 24 months

Secondary outcome measures

Outcome measure	Measure description	Time frame
Change in atrophic lesion size.		From baseline to 24 months.
Maximum Plasma Concentration (Cmax) of Tinlarebant in plasma.		Up to 24 months
Time to Maximum Plasma Concentration (Tmax) of Tinlarebant in plasma.		Up to 24 months
Half-life (t1/2) of Tinlarebant in plasma.		Up to 24 months
Time to minimal plasma RBP4 level (Tmin)		Up to 24 months
Minimum concentration of RBP4 (Cmin)		Up to 24 months

Sponsor
RBP4 Pty Ltd

Collaborators
- Belite Bio, Inc

Investigators
No information provided

General Publications
No publications available

Chapter 6
Completed Studies

United States

The Natural History of the Progression of Atrophy Secondary to Stargardt Disease Type 4: PROM1-Related Macular Dystrophy (ProgStar-4)

ClinicalTrials.gov ID NCT02410122

Sponsor Johns Hopkins University
Information provided by Johns Hopkins University (Responsible Party)
Last Update Posted 2018-08-03

Study Overview

Brief Summary

While a fair amount of clinical data on Stargardt disease type 1 (STGD1) have been published, very little is known about Stargardt disease type 4 (STGD4). The ProgStar 04 study is an important opportunity to leverage the infrastructure, clinical trials sites, methods, and central reading center of the ProgStar program to investigate the progression of STGD4 and will help to establish patient cohorts worldwide for future clinical trials.

Detailed Description

The PROM1 gene codes a protein called Prominin 1 (PROM1; also known as CD133 and AC133), most known for its original use as a human stem cell-specific marker. In the retina, PROM1 is involved in the formation and organization of disks within the outer segment (OS) of the photoreceptors. It is within this particular region that most of the electrochemical signals in response to light are generated (visual cycle-phototransduction). In STGD4, mutations in the PROM1 gene result

J. N. Weiss, *Clinical Trials in Stargardt Disease Treatment*,
https://doi.org/10.1007/978-3-031-58807-5_6

in a defective isoform of the PROM1 protein that becomes trapped in the myoid region of the photoreceptors and cannot migrate to the OS site where disks are formed. Ultimately, the absence of PROM1 in the OS affects the growth and organization of the disks, which leads to disk malfunction and to vision problems.

Although many advances in genetic science have helped to recognize this variant of STGD, a comprehensive description of the natural history, including the variability in cone and rod dysfunction, of this STGD variant is not available. While there is no known treatment for STGD at this time, the preparation for future therapeutic approaches and for planning clinical trials must include an understanding of the disease itself, its variability, its progression, and its correlation with visual loss. Moreover, clinical trials that aim to slow down the progression and/or to restore vision require validated outcome measures to prove treatment efficacy. However, such outcomes have not been established for STGD overall.

In summary, the characterization of STGD4-specific clinical manifestations, progression, and prognosis as well as identification of outcome measures for clinical trials are critical to develop new clinical trials for STGD4. Hence, ProgStar 4 is developed as a prospective longitudinal observational study of patients with mutations in the PROM1 gene and a phenotype consistent with STGD.

Official Title

The Natural History of the Progression of Atrophy Secondary to Stargardt Disease Type 4 (STGD4): A Prospective Longitudinal Observational Study of Stargardt Disease Type4, a PROM1-Related Macular Dystrophy

Conditions

Stargardt Disease

Intervention/Treatment

Other Study ID Numbers

• NA_00092688

Study Start

2014-12

Primary Completion (Actual)

2018-03

Study Completion (Actual)

2018-03

Enrollment (Actual)

15

Study Type

Observational

United States
Maryland Locations

Baltimore, Maryland, United States, 21287

Wilmer Eye Institute

Texas Locations

Dallas, Texas, United States, 75231
Retina Foundation of the Southwest

Germany

Bonn, Germany, 53127
Universitäts-Augenklinik Bonn

Tuebingen, Germany, 72076
Center for Opthalmic Research, University of Tuebingen

United Kingdom

London, United Kingdom, EC1V 2PD
Moorfields Eye Hospital

Eligibility Criteria
Description

Inclusion Criteria
- Provide a signed informed consent form and authorization allowing the disclosure and use of protected health information.
- The designated primary study eye must have at least one well-demarcated area of atrophy. The lesion size should not exceed the area to be tracked in the OCT mode ($20 \times 20°$).
- Have at least one pathogenic mutation confirmed in the PROM1 gene and a Stargardt phenotype.
- The primary study eye must have clear ocular media and adequate pupillary dilation to permit good quality FAF and sd-OCT imaging in the opinion of the investigator.
- Be able to cooperate in performing the examinations.
- Be willing to undergo ocular examinations once every 6 months for up to 24 months.
- Be at least 6 years old.
- Both eyes can be included if inclusion criteria are fulfilled for both eyes.

Exclusion Criteria
- Ocular disease, such as choroidal neovascularization, glaucoma, and diabetic retinopathy, in either eye that may confound assessment of the retina morphologically and functionally.
- Intraocular surgery in the primary study eye within 90 days prior to baseline visit.
- Current or previous participation in an interventional study to treat STGD such as gene therapy or stem cell therapy. Current participation in a drug trial or previous participation in a drug trial within six months before enrollment. The use of oral supplements of vitamins and minerals is permitted, although the current use of Vitamin A supplementation shall be documented.

- The site principal investigator may declare any patient at their site ineligible to participate in the study for a sound medical reason prior to the patient's enrollment into the study.
- Any systemic disease with a limited survival prognosis (e.g., cancer, severe/unstable cardiovascular disease).
- Any condition that would make adherence to the examination interfere with the patient attending their regular follow-up visits schedule of once every 6 months for up to 24 months difficult or unlikely: e.g., personality disorder, use of major tranquilizers such as Haldol or Phenothiazine, chronic alcoholism, Alzheimer's Disease, or drug abuse.
- Evidence of significant uncontrolled concomitant diseases such as cardiovascular, neurological, pulmonary, renal, hepatic, endocrine, or gastrointestinal disorders.
- Patient is known to have one or more pathogenic mutation(s) in the ABCA4, RDS, or ELOVL4 genes.

Study Population

The study shall enroll participants with PROM1 mutations and associated STGD4 phenotype at up to 10 clinical sites.

Ages Eligible for Study

6 Years and older (Child, Adult, Older Adult)

Sexes Eligible for Study

All

Accepts Healthy Volunteers

No

Sampling Method

Non-Probability Sample

Design Details

Observational Model: Cohort

Time Perspective: Prospective

Primary outcome measures

Outcome measure	Measure description	Time frame
Growth of atrophic lesions as measured by fundus autofluorescence (FAF) imaging		24 months

Secondary outcome measures

Outcome measure	Measure description	Time frame
Growth of atrophic lesions as measured by fundus autofluorescence (FAF) imaging		12 months

Outcome measure	Measure description	Time frame
Rate of retinal thinning and photoreceptor loss as measured by spectral-domain optical coherence tomography (sd-OCT)		12 months
Rate of retinal thinning and photoreceptor loss as measured by spectral-domain optical coherence tomography (sd-OCT)		24 months
Loss of retinal sensitivity as measured by microperimetry		12 months
Loss of retinal sensitivity as measured by microperimetry		24 months
Change in best-corrected visual acuity by using the Early-Treatment Diabetic Retinopathy Study (ETDRS) protocol		12 months
Change in best-corrected visual acuity by using the Early-Treatment Diabetic Retinopathy Study (ETDRS) protocol		24 months
Correlation of all outcome measures with genetic profile		12 months
Correlation of all outcome measures with genetic profile		24 months

Sponsor
Johns Hopkins University

Collaborators
- The Shulsky Foundation

Investigators
No information provided

General Publications
No publications available

No Results Posted

United States

Completed

Safety and Efficacy of Emixustat in Stargardt Disease (SeaSTAR)

ClinicalTrials.gov ID NCT03772665

Sponsor Kubota Vision Inc.
Information provided by Kubota Vision Inc. (Responsible Party)
Last Update Posted 2023-08-03

Study Overview

Brief Summary

The purpose of this study is to determine if emixustat hydrochloride reduces the rate of progression of macular atrophy compared to placebo in subjects with Stargardt disease.

Funding Source – FDA OOPD

Detailed Description

Stargardt disease is a rare, inherited degenerative disease of the retina affecting approximately 1 in 8000 to 10 000 people and is the most common type of hereditary macular dystrophy. There are no approved treatments for STGD. This disease is characterized by an excessive accumulation of lipofuscin at the level of the retinal pigment epithelium (RPE). Lipofuscin is made of lipids, proteins, and toxic bis retinoids (such as N retinylidene N retinylethanolamine [A2E]). Accumulation of the toxic bis retinoids found in lipofuscin is thought to cause RPE cell dysfunction and eventual apoptosis, resulting in photoreceptor death and loss of vision.

Stargardt disease has several subtypes, where autosomal recessive STGD (STGD1) accounts for the majority (>95%) of all cases. STGD1 is typically diagnosed in the first 3 decades of life and is caused by mutations of the adenosine triphosphate-binding cassette subfamily A member 4 (ABCA4) gene. The ABCA4 gene product transports N retinylidene phosphatidylethanolamine (a precursor of toxic bis retinoids) from the lumen side of photoreceptor disc membranes to the cytoplasmic side where the retinal is hydrolyzed from phosphatidylethanolamine. Mutations of the ABCA4 gene result in accumulation of this precursor in disc membranes that are eventually phagocytized by RPE cells, where the precursors are converted into toxic bis retinoids such as A2E. In addition to being a precursor to A2E, all trans retinal has also been implicated in the pathogenesis of STGD through its role in light-mediated toxicity.

Emixustat hydrochloride (emixustat) has been developed by Acucela Inc. for retinal diseases including Stargardt disease (STGD). Emixustat is a potent inhibitor of RPE65 isomerization activity and reduces visual chromophore (11 cis-retinal) production in a dose-dependent and reversible manner. Because 11 cis-retinal and its photoproduct (all trans retinal) are substrates for biosynthesis of retinoid toxins (e.g., A2E), chronic treatment with emixustat retards the rate at which these toxins accumulate.

Official Title

A Phase 3 Multicenter, Randomized, Double-Masked Study Comparing the Efficacy and Safety of Emixustat Hydrochloride with Placebo for the Treatment of Macular Atrophy Secondary to Stargardt Disease

Conditions

Stargardt Disease

Intervention/Treatment

- Drug: Emixustat
- Drug: Placebo

Other Study ID Numbers
- 4429-301
- R01FD006849 (U.S. FDA Grant/Contract)

Study Start (Actual)
2018-11-07

Primary Completion (Actual)
2022-06-13

Study Completion (Actual)
2022-06-23

Enrollment (Actual)
194

Study Type
Interventional

Phase
Phase 3

United States
California Locations

Beverly Hills, California, United States, 90211
Retina-Vitreous Associates Medical Group

San Francisco, California, United States, 94143-0730
UCSF Dept. of Ophthalmology

Georgia Locations

Atlanta, Georgia, United States, 30322
Emory University

Maryland Locations

Baltimore, Maryland, United States, 21287
The Wilmer Eye Institute Johns Hopkins University

Michigan Locations

Ann Arbor, Michigan, United States, 48105
University of Michigan Kellogg Eye Center

Minnesota Locations

Rochester, Minnesota, United States, 55905
Mayo Clinic Rochester

North Carolina Locations

Durham, North Carolina, United States, 27710

Duke Eye Center

Oregon Locations

Portland, Oregon, United States, 97239
Casey Eye Institute – OHSU

Texas Locations

Dallas, Texas, United States, 75231
Retina Foundation of the Southwest

Utah Locations

Salt Lake City, Utah, United States, 84132
University of Utah John Moran Eye Center

Wisconsin Locations

Milwaukee, Wisconsin, United States, 53226
Medical College of Wisconsin-Eye Institute

Brazil

São Paulo, Brazil, 04024-002
Hospital Sao Paulo

Minas Gerais Locations

Belo Horizonte, Minas Gerais, Brazil, 30150-320
Santa Casa de Misericórdia de Belo Horizonte

Canada
Ontario Locations

Toronto, Ontario, Canada, MSG 1X8
The Hospital for Sick Children

Denmark
Hovedstaden Locations

Glostrup, Hovedstaden, Denmark, DK-2600
Rigshospitalet-Glostrup

France
Île-de-France Locations

Créteil, Île-de-France, France, 94000
Service D'Ophtalmologie Chi Creteil

Paris, Île-de-France, France, 75012
CHNO Quinze-Vingts – CIC

Germany

Bonn, Germany, 53127
Universitäts-Augenklinik Bonn

Baden-Württemberg Locations

Tübingen, Baden-Württemberg, Germany, 72076
Universitätsklinikum Tübingen, Department für Augenheilkunde

Italy
Campania Locations

Naples, Campania, Italy, 80131
AOU Università della Campania Luigi Vanvitelli

Lazio Locations

Rome, Lazio, Italy, 00168
Università Cattolica del Sacro Cuore—Fondazione Policlinico Gemelli

Lombardy Locations

Milan, Lombardy, Italy, 20132
IRCCS Ospedale San Raffaele

Milan, Lombardy, Italy, 20157
UOC Oculistica Asst Fatebene Pratelli Sacco Universita delgi Studi di Milano

Tuscany Locations

Florence, Tuscany, Italy, 50134
SODC di Oculistica AOU Careggi

Netherlands
Gelderland Locations

Nijmegen, Gelderland, Netherlands, 6500
Radboud University Medical Center

South Africa
Gauteng Locations

Pretoria, Gauteng, South Africa, 0082
Pretoria Eye Institute

Spain

Madrid, Spain, 28040
Fundacion Jimenez Diaz University Hospital

United Kingdom

London, United Kingdom, EC1V 2PD
Moorfields Eye Hospital NHS Foundation Trust

Oxfordshire Locations

Oxford, Oxfordshire, United Kingdom, OXD3 9DU
Oxford Eye Hospital, Oxford University Hospitals NHS Foundation Trust

Eligibility Criteria
Description

Inclusion Criteria
- A clinical diagnosis of macular atrophy secondary to Stargardt disease (STGD)
- Macular atrophy measured to fall within a defined size range
- Two mutations of the ABCA4 gene. If only one mutation, a typical STGD appearance of the retina.
- Visual acuity in the study eye of at least 20/320

Exclusion Criteria
- Macular atrophy secondary to a disease other than STGD
- Mutations of genes, other than ABCA4, that are associated with retinal degeneration
- Surgery in the study eye in the past 3 months
- Prior participation in a gene therapy or stem cell clinical trial for STGD
- Recent participation in a clinical trial for STGD evaluating a complement inhibitor or vitamin A derivative
- Use of certain medications in the past 4 weeks that might interfere with emixustat
- An abnormal electrocardiogram (ECG)
- Certain abnormalities on laboratory blood testing
- Female subjects who are pregnant or nursing

Ages Eligible for Study
16 Years and older (Child, Adult, Older Adult)

Sexes Eligible for Study
All

Accepts Healthy Volunteers
No

Design Details
Primary Purpose: Treatment

Allocation: Randomized

Interventional Model: Parallel Assignment
Interventional Model Description: This is a multicenter, randomized, double-masked, placebo-controlled study to evaluate the efficacy and safety of emixustat compared to placebo in subjects who have macular atrophy secondary to Stargardt disease.

Masking: Quadruple (Participant Care Provider Investigator Outcomes Assessor)
Masking Description: Double-Masked

Arms and interventions

Participant group/arm	Intervention/treatment
Experimental: Emixustat 10 mg	Drug: Emixustat • Once-daily oral tablet taken for 24 months • Other Names: – emixustat hydrochloride
Placebo Comparator: Placebo Includes identical tablets with only inactive ingredients (0 mg).	Drug: Placebo • Once-daily oral tablet taken for 24 months

Primary outcome measures

Outcome measure	Measure description	Time frame
Mean rate of change in total area of macular atrophy, as measured by Fundus Autofluorescence (FAF)	Mean rate of change in total area of macular atrophy, as measured by fundus autofluorescence (FAF)	24 months

Sponsor

Kubota Vision Inc.

Collaborators

• Food and Drug Administration (FDA)

Investigators

• Study Director: Jeff Gregory, MD, VP of Clinical Development, Acucela

General Publications

No publications available

Results

Outcome Measures

1. Mean Rate of Change in Total Area of Macular Atrophy, as Measured by Fundus Autofluorescence (FAF)

Type: Primary|Time Frame: 24 months

Description	Mean rate of change in total area of macular atrophy, as measured by fundus autofluorescence (FAF)
Time Frame	24 months
Analysis Population Description	ITT

Arm/Group Title	Emixustat	Placebo
Arm/Group Description	10 mg Emixustat: Once-daily oral tablet taken for 24 months	Includes identical tablets with only inactive ingredients (0 mg). Placebo: Once-daily oral tablet taken for 24 months Show less
Overall Number of Participants Analyzed	128	66
Mean (Standard Error) | Unit of Measure: Rate of change from BL (mm^2/yr)	1.280(0.0783)	1.309(0.1002)

Adverse Events
Time Frame
24 months
Adverse Event Reporting Description
MedDRA version 25.0

Arm/Group Title	Emixustat	Placebo
Arm/Group Description	10 mg Emixustat: Once-daily oral tablet taken for 24 months	Includes identical tablets with only inactive ingredients (0 mg). Placebo: Once-daily oral tablet taken for 24 months Show more

All-cause mortality

Arm/Group Title	Emixustat	Placebo
	Affected/at Risk (%)	Affected/at Risk (%)
Total	0/127 (0.00%)	0/66 (0.00%)

Serious adverse events

Arm/Group Title	Emixustat		Placebo	
	Affected/at Risk (%)	# Events	Affected/at Risk (%)	# Events
Total	9/127 (7.09%)		2/66 (3.03%)	
Cardiac disorders				
Angina pectoris[a,b]	1/127 (0.79%)	1	1/66 (1.52%)	1
Atrial fibrillation[a,b]	1/127 (0.79%)	1	0/66 (0.00%)	0
Eye disorders				
Visual disorder[a,b]	1/127 (0.79%)	1	0/66 (0.00%)	0
Infections and infestations				
Infections and infestations[a,b]	1/127 (0.79%)	1	1/66 (1.52%)	1
Injury, poisoning, and procedural complications				
Injury, poisoning, and procedural[a,b]	1/127 (0.79%)	1	0/66 (0.00%)	0

Arm/Group Title	Emixustat		Placebo	
Neoplasms benign, malignant, and unspecified (incl cysts and polyps)				
Neoplasm[a,b]	2/127 (1.57%)	2	1/66 (1.52%)	1
Nervous system disorders				
Nervous system disorder[a,b]	1/127 (0.79%)	1	0/66 (0.00%)	0
Vascular disorders				
Vascular disorder[a,b]	1/127 (0.79%)	1	0/66 (0.00%)	0
Other (Not including serious) adverse events				
0% Frequency Threshold for Reporting Other Adverse Events				
Arm/Group Title	Emixustat		Placebo	
	Affected/at Risk (%)	# Events	Affected/at Risk (%)	# Events
Total	1/127 (0.79%)		0/66 (0.00%)	
Eye disorders				
Visual acuity reduced[a,b]	1/127 (0.79%)	1	0/66 (0.00%)	0

[a]Indicates events were collected by systematic assessment
[b]Term from vocabulary, MedDRA 25.0

United States

Completed

A Natural History of the Progression of Stargardt Disease: Retrospective and Prospective Studies (ProgSTAR)

ClinicalTrials.gov ID NCT01977846

Sponsor Foundation Fighting Blindness
Information provided by Foundation Fighting Blindness (Responsible Party)
Last Update Posted 2019-11-01

Study Overview

Brief Summary

Stargardt disease is currently an incurable and untreatable macular dystrophy that causes severe visual loss in children and young adults, thereby causing enormous morbidity with economic, psychological, emotional, and social implications. There are no FDA-approved therapeutic treatments for this disease. Therefore, the objective of this study is to collect natural history data from a large population of children and adults in order to evaluate possible efficacy measures for planned clinical trials.

Participants will be recruited from each investigator's own patient population as the study requires the availability of multiyear retrospective data, as well as ongoing prospectively collected data. A concurrent ancillary study (SMART study) is also being conducted with a subset of the prospective study patients during their regular ProgSTAR study visits to expand the collection of retinal images to include micro-perimetry measurements gathered under scotopic (low light) conditions.

Official Title
Natural History of Progression of Atrophy Secondary to Stargardt Disease: Retrospective and Prospective Longitudinal Observational Study Incl. Ancillary SMART Study-Scotopic Microperimetric Assessment of Rod Function in Stargardt Disease

Conditions
Stargardt Disease

Intervention/Treatment

Other Study ID Numbers
• FFBCRI-PROGSTAR-01/02

Study Start
2013-08

Primary Completion (Actual)
2017-02

Study Completion (Actual)
2017-02

Enrollment (Actual)
259

Study Type
Observational

United States
Maryland Locations

Baltimore, Maryland, United States, 21204
Greater Baltimore Medical Center

Baltimore, Maryland, United States, 21287
Wilmer Eye Institute, Johns Hopkins University

Ohio Locations

Cleveland, Ohio, United States, 44195
Cole Eye Institute, Cleveland Clinic

Pennsylvania Locations

Philadelphia, Pennsylvania, United States, 19104
Scheie Eye Institute, University of Pennsylvania

Texas Locations

Dallas, Texas, United States, 75231
Retina Foundation of the Southwest

Utah Locations

Salt Lake City, Utah, United States, 84132
Moran Eye Center, University of Utah

France

Paris, France, 75012
Institut de la Vision

Germany

Tübingen, Germany, 72076
Center for Ophthalmic Research, University of Teubingen

United Kingdom

London, United Kingdom, EC1V 2PD
Moorfields Eye Hospital

Eligibility Criteria
Description

Inclusion Criteria
- Provide a signed informed consent form and authorization allowing the disclosure and use of protected health information.
- The designated primary study eye must have at least one well-demarcated area of atrophy as imaged by fundus autofluorescence with a minimum diameter of 300 microns and all lesions together must add to less than or equal to 12 mm^2 (equivalent to no more than 5 disc areas in a least one eye) and a BCVA of 20 ETDRS letters (20/400 Snellen equivalent) or better.
- Two (2) pathogenic mutations confirmed present, in the ABCA4 gene. If only one ABCA4 allele contains a pathogenic mutation, the patient shall have a typical Stargardt phenotype, namely at least one eye must have flecks at the level of the retinal pigment epithelium typical for STGD.
- The primary study eye must have clear ocular media and adequate pupillary dilation to permit good quality fundus autofluorescence (FAF) and Spectral-Domain optical coherence tomography (sd-OCT) imaging in the opinion of the investigator.
- Be able to cooperate in performing the examinations.
- Be willing to undergo ocular examinations once every 6 months for up to 24 months.
- Be at least 6 years old.
- Both eyes can be included if inclusion criteria are fulfilled for both eyes.

Exclusion Criteria

- Ocular disease, such as choroidal neovascularization, glaucoma, and diabetic retinopathy, in either eye that may confound assessment of the retina morphologically and functionally.
- Intraocular surgery in the primary study eye within 90 days prior to baseline visit.
- Current or previous participation in an interventional study to treat STGD such as gene therapy or stem cell therapy. Current participation in a drug trial or previous participation in a drug trial within six months before enrollment. The use of oral supplements of vitamins and minerals is permitted, although the current use of Vitamin A supplementation shall be documented.
- The site principal investigator may declare any patient at their site ineligible to participate in the study for a sound medical reason prior to the patient's enrollment into the study.
- Any systemic disease with a limited survival prognosis (e.g., cancer, severe/unstable cardiovascular disease).
- Any condition that would interfere with the patient attending their regular follow-up visits every 6 months for up to 24 months, e.g., personality disorder, use of major tranquilizers such as Haldol or Phenothiazine, chronic alcoholism, Alzheimer's Disease, or drug abuse.
- Evidence of significant uncontrolled concomitant diseases such as cardiovascular, neurological, pulmonary, renal, hepatic, endocrine, or gastrointestinal disorders.

Study Population

The study population shall consist of up to 250 Stargardt disease patients (minimum of 150 patients) recruited at up to 14 clinical centers across the US and Europe. Must be at least 6 years old, able to cooperate in performing the examinations and be willing to attend regular 6-month follow-up visits for up to 24 months. Must present with atrophic lesions secondary to STGD and previously genotyped (at least 2 confirmed pathogenic mutations in the ABCA4 gene). If only 1 ABCA4 allele contains a pathogenic mutation, then the patient needs typical phenotype, i.e., at least one eye must have flecks at the level of the retinal pigment epithelium typical for STGD. Best-corrected visual acuity (BCVA) must be 20 ETDRS letters (20/400 Snellen equivalent) or better.

Ages Eligible for Study

6 Years and older (Child, Adult, Older Adult)

Sexes Eligible for Study

All

Accepts Healthy Volunteers

No

Sampling Method

Non-Probability Sample

Design Details

Observational Model: Case-Only
Time Perspective: Other

Primary outcome measures

Outcome measure	Measure description	Time frame
Yearly progression rate of atrophic lesions using Fundus Autofluorescence (FAF) images	Yearly increase in area of decreased autofluorescence (DAF) which is defined as the sum of definite and questionable decreased autofluorescence	2-12 years

Secondary outcome measures

Outcome measure	Measure description	Time frame
Yearly rate of loss of retinal sensitivity as measured by scotopic microperimetry (MP)	The yearly rate of change in retinal sensitivity. Sensitivity tested with a Nidek MP-1 machine using a modified Humphrey 10-2 grid. The sensitivity was the average sensitivity from a 68-points test pattern (Prospective cohort only)	2 years
Yearly rate of visual acuity loss	Yearly change of visual acuity. Visual acuity measures of best-corrected or presenting VA extracted from medical record charts. Prospective cohort is best-corrected visual acuity using early-treatment diabetic retinopathy study methods	2–12 years
Difference in the rate of retinal sensitivity change per year between photopic and scotopic micro-perimetry testing	Difference in the yearly rate of change in retinal sensitivity under photopic and scotopic conditions. Sensitivity tested with a Nidek MP-1. Scotopic sensitivity was obtained using a 40 points test pattern, and photopic sensitivity was obtained using a 68 points test pattern in a subset of prospective cohort patients	2 years
Yearly rate of loss of overall retinal thickness	Yearly decrease of overall retinal thickness using spectral-domain optical coherence tomography (SD-OCT) scans from a $20° \times 20°$ scan area centered on the fovea. Data are only available for the prospective cohort.	Participants followed at baseline, 6 months, 12 months, and 24 months
Yearly rate of loss of outer ring retinal thickness	Yearly decrease of outer ring retinal thickness using SD-OCT scans from a $20° \times 20°$ scan area centered on the fovea. Outer ring defined as ETDRS fields 1-4.	Participants followed at baseline, 6 months, 12 months, and 24 months

Outcome measure	Measure description	Time frame
Yearly rate of loss of the inner ring retinal thickness	Yearly decrease of the inner ring retinal thickness using SD-OCT scans from a $20° \times 20°$ scan area centered on the fovea. Inner ring defined as ETDRS fields 5-8. Data are only available for the prospective cohort.	Participants followed at baseline, 6 months, 12 months, and 24 months
Yearly rate of loss of the central ring retinal thickness	Yearly decrease of the central ring retinal thickness using SD-OCT scans from a $20° \times 20°$ scan area centered on the fovea. Central area defined as ETDRS fields 9. Data are only available for the prospective cohort.	Participants followed at baseline, 6 months, 12 months, and 24 months

Sponsor
Foundation Fighting Blindness

Collaborators
- United States Department of Defense

Investigators
- Study Chair: Hendrik Scholl, MD, Wilmer Eye Institute at the Johns Hopkins University

General Publications
- Schonbach EM, Ibrahim MA, Strauss RW, Birch DG, Cideciyan AV, Hahn GA, Ho A, Kong X, Nasser F, Sunness JS, Zrenner E, Sadda SR, West SK, Scholl HPN; Progression of Stargardt Disease Study Group. Fixation Location and Stability Using the MP-1 Microperimeter in Stargardt Disease: ProgStar Report No. 3. Ophthalmol Retina. 2017 Jan-Feb;1(1):68–76. https://doi.org/10.1016/j.oret.2016.08.009. Epub 2016 Oct 31.
- Kong X, West SK, Strauss RW, Munoz B, Cideciyan AV, Michaelides M, Ho A, Ahmed M, Schonbach EM, Cheetham JK, Ervin AM, Scholl HPN; ProgStar study group. Progression of Visual Acuity and Fundus Autofluorescence in Recent-Onset Stargardt Disease: ProgStar Study Report #4. Ophthalmol Retina. 2017 Nov-Dec;1(6):514–523. https://doi.org/10.1016/j.oret.2017.02.008. Epub 2017 Apr 28.
- Strauss RW, Munoz B, Ho A, Jha A, Michaelides M, Mohand-Said S, Cideciyan AV, Birch D, Hariri AH, Nittala MG, Sadda S, Scholl HPN; ProgStar Study Group. Incidence of Atrophic Lesions in Stargardt Disease in the Progression of Atrophy Secondary to Stargardt Disease (ProgStar) Study: Report No. 5. JAMA Ophthalmol. 2017 Jul 1;135(7):687–695. https://doi.org/10.1001/jamaophthalmol.2017.1121.
- Schonbach EM, Wolfson Y, Strauss RW, Ibrahim MA, Kong X, Munoz B, Birch DG, Cideciyan AV, Hahn GA, Nittala M, Sunness JS, Sadda SR, West SK, Scholl HPN; ProgStar Study Group. Macular Sensitivity Measured With Microperimetry in Stargardt Disease in the Progression of Atrophy Secondary to Stargardt Disease (ProgStar) Study: Report No. 7. JAMA Ophthalmol. 2017 Jul 1;135(7):696–703. https://doi.org/10.1001/jamaophthalmol.2017.1162.

Results

Outcome Measures

1. Yearly Progression Rate of Atrophic Lesions Using Fundus Autofluorescence (FAF) Images

Type: Primary| Time Frame: 2–12 years

Description	Yearly increase in area of decreased autofluorescence (DAF) which is defined as the sum of definite and questionable decreased autofluorescence
Time Frame	2–12 years
Analysis Population Description	Eyes of participants with at least 2 visits with gradable fundus autofluorescence images with atrophic lesions present

Arm/Group Title	Retrospective Cohort	Prospective Cohort
Arm/Group Description	Subjects with at least two pathogenic mutations in the ABCA4 gene (or one mutation, but the clinical phenotype of flecks at the level of the RPE typical for STGD1). Clinical data from multiple centers extracted from medical records. Participants were to have at least two visits with at least one of the study image modalities (fundus autofluorescence, micro-perimetry, or spectral-domain optical coherence tomography (OCT)) Show more	Multicenter prospective longitudinal cohort. Patients with at least two pathogenic mutations in the ABCA4 gene (or one mutation, but the clinical phenotype of flecks at the level of the RPE typical for STGD1). Participants were to have standardized visits at baseline and every 6 months for 24 months. Participant's data are from clinical examinations and central RC grading of retinal imaging (fundus autofluorescence, spectral-domain optical coherence tomography (OCT)) and micro-perimetry. Show more
Overall number of participants analyzed	215	259
Overall number of units analyzed type of units analyzed: eyes	386	489
Mean (95% Confidence Interval) | Unit of Measure: mm^2/year	0.35(0.28 to 0.43)	0.64(0.57 to 0.71)

2. Yearly Rate of Loss of Retinal Sensitivity as Measured by Scotopic Microperimetry (MP)

Type: Secondary|Time Frame: 2 years

Description	The yearly rate of change in retinal sensitivity. Sensitivity tested with a Nidek MP-1 machine using a modified Humphrey 10-2 grid. The sensitivity was the average sensitivity from a 68-points test pattern (Prospective cohort only)
Time Frame	2 years
Analysis Population Description	Microperimetry data are available for only the prospective cohort at centers with required equipment

Arm/Group Title	Retrospective Cohort	Prospective Cohort
Arm/Group Description	Subjects with at least two pathogenic mutations in the ABCA4 gene (or one mutation, but the clinical phenotype of flecks at the level of the RPE typical for STGD1). Clinical data from multiple centers extracted from medical records. Participants were to have at least two visits with at least one of the study image modalities (fundus autofluorescence, micro-perimetry, or spectral-domain optical coherence tomography (OCT)) Show more	Multicenter prospective longitudinal cohort. Patients with at least two pathogenic mutations in the ABCA4 gene (or one mutation, but the clinical phenotype of flecks at the level of the RPE typical for STGD1). Participants were to have standardized visits at baseline and every 6 months for 24 months. Participant's data are from clinical examinations and central RC grading of retinal imaging (fundus autofluorescence, spectral-domain optical coherence tomography (OCT)) and micro-perimetry. Show more
Overall number of participants analyzed	0	238
Overall number of units analyzed Type of units analyzed: eyes	0	449
Mean (95% Confidence Interval)	Unit of Measure: dB/year		−0.76(−0.87 to −0.66)

3. Yearly Rate of Visual Acuity Loss

Type: Secondary|Time Frame: 2–12 years

Description	Yearly change of visual acuity. Visual acuity measures of best-corrected or presenting VA extracted from medical record charts. Prospective cohort is best-corrected visual acuity using early-treatment diabetic retinopathy study methods
Time Frame	2–12 years
Analysis Population Description	[Not Specified]

Arm/Group Title	Retrospective Cohort	Prospective Cohort
Arm/Group Description	Subjects with at least two pathogenic mutations in the ABCA4 gene (or one mutation, but the clinical phenotype of flecks at the level of the RPE typical for STGD1). Clinical data from multiple centers extracted from medical records. Participants were to have at least two visits with at least one of the study image modalities (fundus autofluorescence, micro-perimetry, or spectral-domain optical coherence tomography (OCT)) Show more	Multicenter prospective longitudinal cohort. Patients with at least two pathogenic mutations in the ABCA4 gene (or one mutation, but the clinical phenotype of flecks at the level of the RPE typical for STGD1). Participants were to have standardized visits at baseline and every 6 months for 24 months. Participant's data are from clinical examinations and central RC grading of retinal imaging (fundus autofluorescence, spectral-domain optical coherence tomography (OCT)) and micro-perimetry. Show more
Overall number of participants analyzed	176	259
Overall number of units analyzed Type of units analyzed: eyes	332	489
Mean (95% Confidence Interval)	Unit of Measure: logMAR/year	0.030(0.026 to 0.043)	0.011(0.004 to 0.018)

4. Difference in the Rate of Retinal Sensitivity Change Per Year Between Photopic and Scotopic Micro-perimetry Testing

Type: Secondary|Time Frame: 2 years

Description	Difference in the yearly rate of change in retinal sensitivity under photopic and scotopic conditions. Sensitivity tested with a Nidek MP-1. Scotopic sensitivity was obtained using a 40 point test pattern, and photopic sensitivity was obtained using a 68 points test pattern in a subset of prospective cohort patients
Time Frame	2 years
Analysis population description	Photopic microperimetry was obtained in a subset of patients, in a single designated study eye

Arm/Group Title	Retrospective Cohort	Prospective Cohort
Arm/Group Description	Subjects with at least two pathogenic mutations in the ABCA4 gene (or one mutation, but the clinical phenotype of flecks at the level of the RPE typical for STGD1). Clinical data from multiple centers extracted from medical records. Participants were to have at least two visits with at least one of the study image modalities (fundus autofluorescence, micro-perimetry, or spectral-domain optical coherence tomography (OCT)) Show more	Multicenter prospective longitudinal cohort. Patients with at least two pathogenic mutations in the ABCA4 gene (or one mutation, but the clinical phenotype of flecks at the level of the RPE typical for STGD1). Participants were to have standardized visits at baseline and every 6 months for 24 months. Participant's data are from clinical examinations and central RC grading of retinal imaging (fundus autofluorescence, spectral-domain optical coherence tomography (OCT)) and micro-perimetry. Show more
Overall number of participants analyzed	0	118
Overall number of units analyzed Type of units analyzed: eyes	0	118
Mean (95% Confidence Interval)	Unit of Measure: dB/year		−0.78(−1.16 to −0.41)

5. Yearly Rate of Loss of Overall Retinal Thickness

Type: Secondary|Time Frame: Participants followed at baseline, 6 months, 12 months, and 24 months

Description	Yearly decrease of overall retinal thickness using spectral-domain optical coherence tomography (SD-OCT) scans from a 20° × 20° scan area centered on the fovea. Data are only available for the prospective cohort.
Time Frame	Participants followed at baseline, 6 months, 12 months, and 24 months
Analysis population description	All visits of eligible eyes of the 258 participants with gradable overall thickness. Only OCT scans with adequate and fair quality are included

Arm/Group Title	Prospective Cohort
Arm/Group Description	Multicenter prospective longitudinal cohort. Patients with at least two pathogenic mutations in the ABCA4 gene (or one mutation, but the clinical phenotype of flecks at the level of the RPE typical for STGD1). OCT scans were graded by a central reading center.
Overall number of participants analyzed	258
Overall number of units analyzed Type of units analyzed: eyes	487
Mean (95% Confidence Interval) | Unit of Measure: microns/year	−2.85(−3.19 to −2.52)

6. Yearly Rate of Loss of Outer Ring Retinal Thickness

Type: Secondary|Time Frame: Participants followed at baseline, 6 months, 12 months, and 24 months

Description	Yearly decrease of outer ring retinal thickness using SD-OCT scans from a 20° × 20° scan area centered on the fovea. Outer ring defined as ETDRS fields 1-4.
Time Frame	Participants followed at baseline, 6 months, 12 months, and 24 months
Analysis population description	All visits of eligible eyes of the 258 participants with gradable thickness in the outer ring. Only OCT scans with adequate and fair quality are included

Arm/Group Title	Prospective Cohort
Arm/Group Description	Multicenter prospective longitudinal cohort. Patients with at least two pathogenic mutations in the ABCA4 gene (or one mutation, but the clinical phenotype of flecks at the level of the RPE typical for STGD1). OCT scans were graded by a central reading center.
Overall number of participants analyzed	258

Arm/Group Title	Prospective Cohort
Overall number of units analyzed Type of units analyzed: eyes	487
Mean (95% Confidence Interval) | Unit of Measure: microns/year	−2.84 (−3.19 to −2.50)

7. Yearly Rate of Loss of the Inner Ring Retinal Thickness

Type: Secondary|Time Frame: Participants followed at baseline, 6 months, 12 months, and 24 months

Description	Yearly decrease of the inner ring retinal thickness using SD-OCT scans from a 20° × 20° scan area centered on the fovea. Inner ring defined as ETDRS fields 5–8. Data are only available for the prospective cohort.
Time Frame	Participants followed at baseline, 6 months, 12 months, and 24 months
Analysis Population Description	All visits of eligible eyes of the 258 participants with gradable thickness in the inner ring. Only OCT scans with adequate and fair quality are included

Arm/Group Title	Prospective Cohort
Arm/Group Description	Multicenter prospective longitudinal cohort. Patients with at least two pathogenic mutations in the ABCA4 gene (or one mutation, but the clinical phenotype of flecks at the level of the RPE typical for STGD1). OCT scans were graded by a central reading center.
Overall number of participants analyzed	258
Overall number of units analyzed Type of units analyzed: eyes	487
Mean (95% Confidence Interval) | Unit of Measure: microns/year	−3.20(−3.68 to −2.72)

8. Yearly Rate of Loss of the Central Ring Retinal Thickness

Type: Secondary|Time Frame: Participants followed at baseline, 6 months, 12 months, and 24 months

Description	Yearly decrease of the central ring retinal thickness using SD-OCT scans from a 20° × 20° scan area centered on the fovea. Central area defined as ETDRS fields 9. Data are only available for the prospective cohort.
Time Frame	Participants followed at baseline, 6 months, 12 months, and 24 months
Analysis population description	All visits of eligible eyes of the 258 participants with gradable thickness in the inner ring. Only OCT scans with adequate and fair quality are included

Arm/Group Title	Prospective Cohort
Arm/Group Description	Multicenter prospective longitudinal cohort. Patients with at least two pathogenic mutations in the ABCA4 gene (or one mutation, but the clinical phenotype of flecks at the level of the RPE typical for STGD1). OCT scans were graded by a central reading center.
Overall number of participants analyzed	258
Overall number of units analyzed Type of units analyzed: eyes	487
Mean (95% Confidence Interval) | Unit of Measure: microns/year	−2.24(−3.06 to −1.42)

Adverse Events
Time Frame
Adverse events were not collected in this natural history study
Adverse Event Reporting Description
As there was no intervention in this study, adverse events were not collected

Arm/Group Title	Retrospective Cohort	Prospective Cohort
Arm/Group Description	Subjects with at least two pathogenic mutations in the ABCA4 gene (or one mutation, but the clinical phenotype of flecks at the level of the RPE typical for STGD1). Clinical data from multiple centers extracted from medical records. Participants should had at least two visits with at least one of the study image modalities (fundus autofluorescence, micro-perimetry, or spectral-domain optical coherence tomography (OCT)). Adverse events were not collected Show m	

Arm/Group Title	Retrospective Cohort	Prospective Cohort
Arm/Group Description	Subjects with at least two pathogenic mutations in the ABCA4 gene (or one mutation, but the clinical phenotype of flecks at the level of the RPE typical for STGD1). Clinical data from multiple centers extracted from medical records. Participants should have had at least two visits with at least one of the study image modalities (fundus autofluorescence, micro-perimetry, or spectral-domain optical coherence tomography (OCT)). Adverse events were not collected Show less	Multicenter prospective longitudinal cohort. Patients with at least two pathogenic mutations in the ABCA4 gene (or one mutation, but the clinical phenotype of flecks at the level of the RPE typical for STGD1). Participants had standardized visits at baseline and every 6 months for 24 months. Participant's data are from clinical examinations and central RC grading of retinal imaging (fundus autofluorescence, spectral-domain optical coherence tomography (OCT)) and micro-perimetry. Adverse events were not collected Show less

Arm/Group Title	Retrospective Cohort	Prospective Cohort
All-cause mortality		
Arm/Group Title	Retrospective Cohort	Prospective Cohort
	Affected/at Risk (%)	Affected/at Risk (%)
Total	0/251 (0.00%)	1/259 (0.39%)
Serious adverse events		
Arm/Group Title	Retrospective Cohort	Prospective Cohort
	Affected/at Risk (%)	Affected/at Risk (%)
Total	0/0	0/0
Other (Not including serious) adverse events		
0% Frequency Threshold for Reporting Other Adverse Events		
Arm/Group Title	Retrospective Cohort	Prospective Cohort
	Affected/at Risk (%)	Affected/at Risk (%)
Total	0/0	0/0

United States

Completed

Study of STG-001 in Subjects with Stargardt Disease

ClinicalTrials.gov ID NCT04489511

Sponsor Stargazer Pharmaceuticals, Inc.
Information provided by Stargazer Pharmaceuticals, Inc. (Responsible Party)
Last Update Posted 2021-04-27

Study Overview

Brief Summary

This is an open-label, multicenter study in subjects with Stargardt disease, comparing 2 doses of STG-001 with regard to safety, pharmacokinetics, and pharmacodynamics.

Detailed Description

This is an open-label, multicenter, active treatment study in approximately 12 subjects aged 18 to 55 years (inclusive) with STGD1, genotyped with a minimum of two ABCA4 gene mutations. Treatment course of STG-001 at Dose 1 (Cohort 1) or Dose 2 (Cohort 2) testing doses will be administered once daily for 28 days. Cohorts will run in parallel. Subjects will receive their designated dose daily for 28 days and be monitored for safety measures during the dosing period and for an additional 28 days after dosing (through Day 56).

Official Title
A Phase 2a Study of the Safety, Pharmacokinetics, and Pharmacodynamics of STG-001 in Subjects with Stargardt Disease (STGD1) Caused by Autosomal Recessive Mutation in ATP-Binding Cassette Subfamily A Member 4 (ABCA4) Gene

Conditions
Stargardt Disease-1

Intervention/Treatment
- Drug: STG-001

Other Study ID Numbers
- STG-001-2a

Study Start (Actual)
2020-10-01

Primary Completion (Actual)
2021-04-24

Study Completion (Actual)
2021-04-24

Enrollment (Actual)
10

Study Type
Interventional

Phase
Phase 2

United States
Arizona Locations

Phoenix, Arizona, United States, 85020
Associated Retina Consultants

Florida Locations

Gainesville, Florida, United States, 32607
Vitreo Retinal Associates, P.A.

Oregon Locations

Portland, Oregon, United States, 97239
Casey Eye Institute—OHSU

Pennsylvania Locations

Pittsburgh, Pennsylvania, United States, 15213
UPMC Eye Center

Texas Locations

Dallas, Texas, United States, 75231
Retina Foundation of Southwest

Eligibility Criteria
Description

Inclusion Criteria
- Understand the study procedures and agree to participate by providing written informed consent.
- STGD1 caused by autosomal recessive mutation in the ABCA4 gene (i.e., at least 2 mutations), confirmed genotypically by a fully accredited certified central genotyping laboratory.
- 18–55 years of age inclusive.
- Negative pregnancy testing for women of childbearing potential and highly effective double barrier contraception before, during, and for a period after study treatment as described in the clinical protocol.
- Primary study eye must have at least one well-demarcated area of significantly reduced autofluorescence as imaged by fundus autofluorescence (FAF)
- In at least one eye and in the same eye:

    - ETDRS BCVA of less than or equal to 0.4 logMAR ($\leq$68 letters; 20/50 Snellen equivalent) and greater than or equal to 1.3 logMAR ($\geq$19 letters; 20/400 Snellen equivalent); and
    - Clinical evidence of a macular lesion phenotypically consistent with Stargardt Disease

- Naïve to investigational treatment for STGD1 with no history of gene therapy, stem cell therapy, surgical implantation of prosthetic retinal chips, or intravitreal or subretinal injections. History of experimental oral therapy is allowed if it occurred greater than 3 months prior to screening.
- Primary study eye must have clear ocular media and adequate pupillary dilation, including no allergy to dilating eyedrops, to permit good quality retinal imaging.
- In good general health, aside from STGD1, as judged by investigator.
- Willing and able to comply with the protocol, including attending assessment visits.

Exclusion Criteria
- The subject is an employee of the sponsor or study site or immediate family member (e.g., spouse, parent, child, sibling) of the sponsor or study site.
- Use of prescription or nonprescription drugs and dietary supplements within 7 days or 5 half-lives (whichever is longer) prior to Day 1 first dose. Herbal supplements and HRT must be discontinued 7 days prior to Day 1 first dose.
- Presence of any concurrent ocular disease that would affect study outcomes (e.g., severe cataracts; subjects can be enrolled 3 months after successful cataract surgery).

- Presence of any meaningful retinopathy/maculopathy/atrophy other than as a result of STGD1 in either eye as determined by the investigator.
- Has taken non-approved items (supplement containing vitamin A or beta-carotene, liver-based products, or prescription oral retinoid medications) within 30 days of screening.
- Use of medications that may interact with Vitamin A metabolism within 60 days of screening.
- Participation in an oral interventional study of a vitamin A derivative up to 3 months prior to screening.
- The subject had a history of vitamin A deficiency as defined based upon serum values less than 20 mcg/dl (0.7 μmol/L) or clinical signs during slit-lamp examination (conjunctival or corneal xerosis; Bitot's spots; corneal ulcers or scarring not due to trauma or other secondary causes).
- Presence of significant cardiovascular or cerebrovascular disease, including stroke, within 12 months of entry.
- Has a clinically significant abnormal electrocardiogram (ECG) or has a corrected QT interval (QTc) that is 450 ms or greater.
- Resting heart rate outside specified limits (< 40/min, > 100/min) upon repeated measurement.
- History of diabetes, hepatitis, pancreatitis, cirrhosis, liver failure, uncontrolled thyroid disease, or hypervitaminosis A.
- Any intraocular surgery or thermal laser within 3 months of trial entry. Any prior thermal laser in the macular region.
- Any major surgical procedure within one month of screening or planned or anticipated surgery during the study period.
- Women who are pregnant, nursing, or planning to become pregnant during the study period.
- Uncontrolled blood pressure outside specified limits (90 mm Hg > Systolic > 140 mm Hg and/or 40 mm Hg > Diastolic > 90 mm Hg) upon repeated measurement.
- Clinically significant abnormal lab results at screening, including liver function test (aspartate transaminase, alanine transaminase, bilirubin, and alkaline phosphatase) greater than 1.5 x the upper limit of normal (ULN).
- Actively participating in an investigational therapy study or have received any investigational therapy within 60 days of screening or 5 half-lives, whichever is longer.
- Known serious allergies to the fluorescein dye used to measure intraocular pressure, ocular dilating drops, topical ocular anesthetic, components of the STG-001 formulation, or any history of anaphylaxis reaction.
- In the investigator's assessment, any acute or chronic medical condition, psychiatric condition, physical examination finding, or laboratory abnormality that might increase the risk associated with study participation or administration of study treatment or interfere with the interpretation of study results.

Ages Eligible for Study
18–55 Years (Adult)

Sexes Eligible for Study
All

Accepts Healthy Volunteers
No

Design Details
Primary Purpose: Treatment
Allocation: Non-Randomized
Interventional Model: Parallel Assignment
Masking: None (Open Label)

Arms and interventions

Participant group/arm	Intervention/treatment
Experimental: Dose 1 STG-001 given orally at Dose 1 once a day for 28 days	Drug: STG-001 • Dose 1 or Dose 2 of STG-001 will be administered daily for 28 days to compare safety, pharmacokinetics, and pharmacodynamics in Stargardt disease subjects.
Experimental: Dose 2 STG-001 given orally at Dose 2 once a day for 28 days	Drug: STG-001 • Dose 1 or Dose 2 of STG-001 will be administered daily for 28 days to compare safety, pharmacokinetics, and pharmacodynamics in Stargardt disease subjects.

Primary outcome measures

Outcome measure	Measure description	Time frame
Safety events and tolerability of STG-001 from baseline to 28 days: adverse events	Safety and tolerability of 28 days of daily dosing of 2 doses of STG-001 assessed by incidence and/or clinically significant changes of a combination of ocular and non-ocular adverse events	From baseline to 28 days

Secondary outcome measures

Outcome measure	Measure description	Time frame
Pharmacokinetics (PK) of STG-001 maximum plasma concentration (Cmax) at Day 28	Cmax of 2 doses of STG-001 after 28 days of daily dosing of STG-001 assessed by a validated STG-001 assay	From baseline to 28 days
Pharmacokinetics (PK) of STG-001 area under the curve (AUC) at Day 28	Exposure to STG-001 as assessed by calculated AUC of 2 doses of STG-001 after 28 days of daily dosing of STG-001	From baseline to 28 days
Pharmacodynamics (PD) of STG-001 change in plasma Retinol-Binding Protein 4 (RBP4) at Day 28	Change in Plasma RBP4 levels from baseline to Day 28 with 2 doses of STG-001 after 28 days of daily dosing of STG-001	From baseline to 28 days

Sponsor
Stargazer Pharmaceuticals, Inc.

Collaborators
No information provided

Investigators
- Principal Investigator: Principal Investigator, MD, Study Site Director

General Publications
No publications available

Results Overview
Results Submitted—Quality Control Review Has Not Concluded

United States

Completed

DHA Supplementation in Patients With STGD3

ClinicalTrials.gov ID NCT00420602

Sponsor University of Utah
Information provided by Paul S. Bernstein, University of Utah (Responsible Party)
Last Update Posted 2018-05-09

Study Overview

Brief Summary
We have found that biomarkers of long-term elevated dietary intake of omega-3
fatty acids such as DHA and EPA are inversely associated with severity of disease
phenotype in STGD3 patients. Therefore, the purpose of this study is to follow
STGD3 patients as they supplement their diets with DHA/EPA.

Official Title
Clinical Interventions Against Stargardt Macular Dystrophy: DHA Supplementation
   in Patients with STGD3

Conditions
Dominantly Inherited Stargardt's Disease (STGD3)

Intervention/Treatment
- Dietary Supplement: Over-the-counter DHA/EPA dietary supplementation

Other Study ID Numbers
IRB 19676

Study Start (Actual)
2007-09-21

Primary Completion (Actual)
2017-12-27

Study Completion (Actual)
2017-12-27

Enrollment (Actual)
11

Study Type
Interventional

Phase
Not Applicable

United States
Utah Locations

Salt Lake City, Utah, United States, 84132
Moran Eye Center, University of Utah

Eligibility Criteria
Description

Inclusion Criteria
- All Moran Eye Center patients with STGD3

Exclusion Criteria
- All others

Ages Eligible for Study
18–105 Years (Adult, Older Adult)

Sexes Eligible for Study
All

Accepts Healthy Volunteers
No

Design Details
Primary Purpose: Prevention
Allocation: N/A
Interventional Model: Single Group Assignment
Masking: None (Open Label)

Arms and interventions

Participant group/arm	Intervention/treatment
Other: Single-arm, open-label single-arm, Open Label	Dietary Supplement: Over-the-counter DHA/EPA dietary supplementation • 1000 mg/day DHA/EPA

Primary outcome measures

Outcome measure	Measure description	Time frame
ERG		1 year

Secondary outcome measures

Outcome measure	Measure description	Time frame
Visual acuity		1 year

Sponsor
University of Utah

Collaborators
No information provided

Investigators
• Principal Investigator: Paul S. Bernstein, MD Ph.D., University of Utah

General Publications
No publications available

No Results Posted

United States

Completed

Pharmacodynamic Study of Emixustat Hydrochloride in Subjects with Macular Atrophy Secondary to Stargardt Disease

ClinicalTrials.gov ID NCT03033108

Sponsor Kubota Vision Inc.
Information provided by Kubota Vision Inc. (Responsible Party)
Last Update Posted 2021-05-19

Study Overview

Brief Summary
This is a pharmacodynamics study of Emixustat Hydrochloride in subjects with macular atrophy secondary to Stargardt disease.

Detailed Description
This is a multicenter, randomized, masked study to characterize the pharmacodynamics, safety, and tolerability of emixustat in subjects with macular atrophy secondary to Stargardt disease.

Official Title

A Phase 2a Multicenter, Randomized, Masked Study Evaluating the Pharmacodynamics of Emixustat Hydrochloride in Subjects with Macular Atrophy Secondary to Stargardt Disease

Conditions

Stargardt Disease
Macular Atrophy

Intervention/Treatment

- Drug: Emixustat

Other Study ID Numbers

- 4429-204

Study Start (Actual)

2017-01

Primary Completion (Actual)

2017-11

Study Completion (Actual)

2017-12

Enrollment (Actual)

23

Study Type

Interventional

Phase

Phase 2

United States
Texas Locations

Dallas, Texas, United States, 75231

Eligibility Criteria
Description

Inclusion Criteria, Including, but not Limited to

- Clinical diagnosis of macular atrophy (MA) secondary to Stargardt disease (STGD) in one or both eyes
- At least 2 pathogenic mutations of the ABCA4 gene
- Early-Treatment Diabetic Retinopathy Study BCVA of $\geq$ 20 letters (approximately $\geq$ 20/400 Snellen) in the study eye
- Adequate clarity of ocular media and adequate pupillary dilation to permit good quality imaging of MA in the study eye
- Able and willing to provide written informed consent before undergoing any study-related procedures
- Able to reliably administer oral medication by self or with available assistance

Exclusion Criteria, Including, but not Limited to

- Macular atrophy associated with a condition other than STGD in either eye.
- Presence in either eye of an active ocular disease that in the opinion of the investigator compromises or confounds visual function.
- History of any intraocular or ocular surface surgery in either eye within 3 months of screening.
- Current or previous participation in an interventional study to treat STGD using gene therapy or stem cell therapy at any time, or participation in an interventional study of a vitamin A derivative ≤ 3 months prior to screening.
- Prespecified laboratory abnormalities at screening
- Presence of other medical or ophthalmic disease, physical examination finding, or clinical laboratory finding that in the opinion of the investigator may contraindicate the use of an investigational drug and place the subject at risk
- Current or history of cancer (except for adequately treated basal cell or squamous cell carcinoma of the skin) within 1 year of screening
- History of myocardial infarction, stroke, unstable ischemic heart disease, uncontrolled cardiac arrhythmia, or hospitalization for congestive heart failure within 6 months of screening.
- Anticipated hospitalization for a medical/surgical procedure(s) that could result in interruption/premature cessation of study treatment or participation.
- Electrocardiogram with a clinically significant abnormal finding
- Female subjects who are pregnant or lactating
- Female subjects of childbearing potential or male subjects who are not surgically sterile who are not willing to practice a medically accepted method of birth control with their sexual partner from screening through 30 days after the final dose of study drug.

Ages Eligible for Study
18 Years and older (Adult, Older Adult)

Sexes Eligible for Study
All

Accepts Healthy Volunteers
No

Design Details
Primary Purpose: Treatment
Allocation: Randomized
Interventional Model: Parallel Assignment
Masking: Quadruple (Participant Care Provider Investigator Outcomes Assessor)

Arms and interventions

Participant group/arm	Intervention/treatment
Experimental: Emixustat Dose 1 lowest dose of once-daily oral Emixustat	Drug: Emixustat • Once-daily, tablet for oral administration • Other Names: – Emixustat Hydrochloride

Participant group/arm	Intervention/treatment
Experimental: Emixustat Dose 2 middle dose of once-daily oral Emixustat	Drug: Emixustat • Once-daily, tablet for oral administration • Other Names: – Emixustat Hydrochloride
Experimental: Emixustat Dose 3 highest dose of once-daily oral Emixustat	Drug: Emixustat • Once-daily, tablet for oral administration • Other Names: – Emixustat Hydrochloride

Primary outcome measures

Outcome measure	Measure description	Time frame
Change in electrical response of the retina to a flash of light, as measured by electroretinogram	Percent suppression compared to baseline of rod b-wave amplitude recovery after a photobleaching light.	Baseline and 1 month

Secondary outcome measures

Outcome measure	Measure description	Time frame
Percentage of subjects with adverse events, by severity and seriousness	Assessment of safety profile	1 month

Sponsor
Kubota Vision Inc.

Collaborators
No information provided

Investigators
• Study Director: Acucela Medical Director, MD, Kubota Vision Inc.

General Publications
No publications available

Results

Outcome Measures

1. Change in Electrical Response of the Retina to a Flash of Light, as Measured by Electroretinogram

Type: Primary|Time Frame: Baseline and 1 month

Description	Percent suppression compared to baseline of rod b-wave amplitude recovery after a photobleaching light.
Time Frame	Baseline and 1 month
Analysis population description	Subjects with evaluable ERGs at both Baseline and Month 1

Arm/Group Title	Emixustat Dose 1	Emixustat Dose 2	Emixustat Dose 3
Arm/Group Description	lowest dose of once-daily oral Emixustat Emixustat: Once-daily, tablet for oral administration Show less	middle dose of once-daily oral Emixustat Emixustat: Once-daily, tablet for oral administration Show less	highest dose of once-daily oral Emixustat Emixustat: Once-daily, tablet for oral administration Show less
Overall number of participants analyzed	6	7	6
Median (Full Range)	Unit of Measure: percent suppression	−12.23(−41.0 to 54.7)	68.00(1.0 to 91.5)	96.69(64.9 to 100.0)

2. Percentage of Subjects with Adverse Events, by Severity and Seriousness

Type: Secondary|Time Frame: 1 month

Description	Assessment of safety profile
Time Frame	1 month
Analysis Population Description	[Not Specified]

Arm/Group Title	Emixustat Dose 1	Emixustat Dose 2	Emixustat Dose 3
Arm/Group Description	lowest dose of once-daily oral Emixustat Emixustat: Once-daily, tablet for oral administration Show more	middle dose of once-daily oral Emixustat Emixustat: Once-daily, tablet for oral administration Show more	highest dose of once-daily oral Emixustat Emixustat: Once-daily, tablet for oral administration Show more
Overall number of participants analyzed	7	9	7
Subjects with 1 or more adverse events	685.7%	888.9%	685.7%
Subjects with 1 or more mild adverse events[a]	571.4%	555.6%	457.1%
Subjects with 1 or more moderate adverse events[a]	114.3%	222.2%	228.6%

Arm/Group Title	Emixustat Dose 1	Emixustat Dose 2	Emixustat Dose 3
Subjects with 1 or more severe adverse events[a]	00.0%	111.1%	114.3%
Subjects with 1 or more serious adverse events[a]	00.0%	00.0%	00.0%

[a]Measure Type: Count of Participants | Unit of Measure: Participants

Adverse Events
Time Frame
1 month

Arm/Group Title	Emixustat Dose 1	Emixustat Dose 2	Emixustat Dose 3
Arm/Group Description	lowest dose of once-daily oral Emixustat Emixustat: Once-daily, tablet for oral administration Show more	middle dose of once-daily oral Emixustat Emixustat: Once-daily, tablet for oral administration Show more	highest dose of once-daily oral Emixustat Emixustat: Once-daily, tablet for oral administration Show more

All-cause mortality

Arm/Group Title	Emixustat Dose 1	Emixustat Dose 2	Emixustat Dose 3
	Affected/at Risk (%)	Affected/at Risk (%)	Affected/at Risk (%)
Total	0/7 (0.00%)	0/9 (0.00%)	0/7 (0.00%)

Serious adverse events

Arm/Group Title	Emixustat Dose 1	Emixustat Dose 2	Emixustat Dose 3
	Affected/at Risk (%)	Affected/at Risk (%)	Affected/at Risk (%)
Total	0/7 (0.00%)	0/9 (0.00%)	0/7 (0.00%)

Other (Not including serious) adverse events

5% Frequency Threshold for Reporting Other Adverse Events

Arm/Group Title	Emixustat Dose 1	Emixustat Dose 2	Emixustat Dose 3
	Affected/at Risk (%)	Affected/at Risk (%)	Affected/at Risk (%)
Total	6/7 (85.71%)	8/9 (88.89%)	7/7 (100.00%)
Eye disorders			
Delayed dark adaptation[a,b]	1/7 (14.29%)	6/9 (66.67%)	4/7 (57.14%)
Erythropsia[a,b]	1/7 (14.29%)	3/9 (33.33%)	1/7 (14.29%)
Vision blurred[a,b]	2/7 (28.57%)	1/9 (11.11%)	1/7 (14.29%)
Photophobia[a,b]	1/7 (14.29%)	2/9 (22.22%)	0/7 (0.00%)
Visual impairment[a,b]	1/7 (14.29%)	1/9 (11.11%)	1/7 (14.29%)
Blindness day[a,b]	0/7 (0.00%)	1/9 (11.11%)	1/7 (14.29%)
Chromatopsia[a,b]	0/7 (0.00%)	0/9 (0.00%)	2/7 (28.57%)
Night blindness[a,b]	0/7 (0.00%)	1/9 (11.11%)	1/7 (14.29%)
Xanthopsia[a,b]	0/7 (0.00%)	1/9 (11.11%)	1/7 (14.29%)
Asthenopia[a,b]	1/7 (14.29%)	0/9 (0.00%)	0/7 (0.00%)

Arm/Group Title	Emixustat Dose 1	Emixustat Dose 2	Emixustat Dose 3
Eye Pain[a,b]	1/7 (14.29%)	0/9 (0.00%)	0/7 (0.00%)
Eye Pruritis[a,b]	1/7 (14.29%)	0/9 (0.00%)	0/7 (0.00%)
Lenticular opacities[a,b]	0/7 (0.00%)	0/9 (0.00%)	1/7 (14.29%)
Visual acuity reduced[a,b]	0/7 (0.00%)	0/9 (0.00%)	1/7 (14.29%)
Infections and infestations			
Upper respiratory tract infections[a,b]	0/7 (0.00%)	1/9 (11.11%)	0/7 (0.00%)
Investigations			
Blood bilirubin increased[a,b]	0/7 (0.00%)	1/9 (11.11%)	1/7 (14.29%)
Blood creatine phosphokinase increased[a,b]	0/7 (0.00%)	1/9 (11.11%)	1/7 (14.29%)
Nervous system disorders			
Headache[a,b]	0/7 (0.00%)	2/9 (22.22%)	2/7 (28.57%)
Visual field defect[a,b]	1/7 (14.29%)	0/9 (0.00%)	0/7 (0.00%)
Respiratory, thoracic, and mediastinal disorders			
Cough[a,b]	1/7 (14.29%)	0/9 (0.00%)	0/7 (0.00%)
Rhinorrheoea[a,b]	1/7 (14.29%)	0/9 (0.00%)	0/7 (0.00%)
Skin and subcutaneous tissue disorders			
Dermatitis allergic[a,b]	0/7 (0.00%)	1/9 (11.11%)	0/7 (0.00%)
Rash[a,b]	0/7 (0.00%)	1/9 (11.11%)	0/7 (0.00%)

[a]Indicates events were collected by systematic assessment
[b]Term from vocabulary, MedDRA 20.1

United States

Completed

Microcurrent Stimulation to Treat Macular Degeneration

ClinicalTrials.gov ID NCT01790958

Sponsor Retina Institute of Hawaii
Information provided by Retina Institute of Hawaii (Responsible Party)
Last Update Posted 2013-02-13

Study Overview

Brief Summary
Microcurrent stimulation therapy improves retinal efficiency and may restore and/or improve retinal function.

Detailed Description

This is an observational study in which data will be collected from a group of patients with retinal diseases such as Dry Macular Degeneration, Retinitis Pigmentosa, and Stargardt's Disease, who have opted to receive Microcurrent Stimulation Therapy as an alternative treatment for their retinal condition.

Official Title

An Observational, Multicenter Phase 1 Study of the Safety and Effectiveness of Frequency-Specific Microcurrent Stimulation as an Alternative Treatment for Retinal Diseases

Conditions

Retinal Diseases
Stargardt's Disease
Retinitis Pigmentosa

Intervention/Treatment

Other Study ID Numbers
- RIH 1009

Study Start
2012-06

Primary Completion (Actual)
2012-12

Study Completion (Actual)
2012-12

Enrollment (Actual)
50

Study Type
Observational

United States
Hawaii Locations

Hilo, Hawaii, United States, 96720
Hawaii Cataract Laser Institute—Hilo

Honolulu, Hawaii, United States, 96815
Retina Institute of Hawaii

Kahului, Hawaii, United States, 96732
Hawaii Cataract Laser Institute—Maui

Kailua-Kona, Hawaii, United States, 96740
Hawaii Cataract Laser Institute—Kona

Eligibility Criteria
Description

Inclusion Criteria
- Ability to provide written consent and comply with follow-up visits
- Age 40 years or older
- ETDRS best-corrected visual acuity better than 5 letters
- History of Dry Age-Related Macular Degeneration; Retinitis Pigmentosa; Stargardt's disease
- No Anti-VEGF treatments for at least 3 months prior to study
- No new antioxidant/vitamin supplementation for at least 3 months prior to study

Exclusion Criteria
- History of noncompliance with regular medical visits
- Significant media opacities (exclude NS 4+) that may interfere with assessing visual acuity
- Presence of pigment epithelial tears or rips
- Known serious allergies to fluorescein dye
- Presence of retinal neovascularization
- Any treatment with an investigation agent in the past 30 days

Study Population
Patients with retinal disease such as Age-Related Macular Degeneration, Stargardt's Disease, and Retinitis Pigmentosa

Ages Eligible for Study
50 Years and older (Adult, Older Adult)

Sexes Eligible for Study
All

Accepts Healthy Volunteers
Yes
Sampling Method
Non-Probability Sample

Design Details
Observational Model: Case-Control
Time Perspective: Retrospective

Primary outcome measures

Outcome measure	Measure description	Time frame
Measure visual acuity after receiving microcurrent stimulation treatments.		6 months

Sponsor
Retina Institute of Hawaii

Collaborators
No information provided

Investigators
- Principal Investigator: George Papastergiou, MD, Retina Institute of Hawaii

General Publications
No publications available

United States

Completed

Phase 1 Pilot Study of 4-MP to Treat Stargardt Macular Dystrophy

ClinicalTrials.gov ID NCT00346853

Sponsor University of Utah
Information provided by University of Utah
Last Update Posted 2020-08-05

Study Overview

Brief Summary
The purpose of this study is to investigate whether taking 4-methylpyrazole (4-MP, fomepizole, Antizol™) inhibits dark adaptation of the eye. In other words, we are testing if 4-MP slows the processing of vitamin A derivatives in the eye. By slowing down these processes, individuals with Stargardt disease may have better chances of saving their remaining vision. 4-MP has been shown to slow dark adaptation in animals and is FDA-approved for human use to treat individuals with methanol or ethylene glycol (antifreeze) poisoning by shutting down the body's ability to process alcohols. This medication has an excellent safety profile and has been reported to have no short-term or long-term side effects, as long as patients refrain from any alcohol while the medication is in the body. A single dose of 4-MP remains in the body for about 12 h, and therefore, it may inhibit dark adaptation of your eyes for up to 12 h. Studying the effects of 4-MP may lead to effective medical treatment to save Stargardt patients' vision and may also have similar effects in other macular degenerative diseases.

Official Title
Clinical Interventions Against Stargardt Macular Dystrophy: Phase 1 Pilot Study of 4-MP as an Inhibitor of Dark Adaptation

Conditions
Macular Dystrophy, Corneal

Intervention/Treatment
- Drug: 4-Methylpyrazole
- Other: saline

Other Study ID Numbers
- 4-MP Dark Adaptation Inhib.

Study Start
2005-11

Primary Completion (Actual)
2006-05

Study Completion (Actual)
2006-09

Enrollment (Actual)
10

Study Type
Interventional

Phase
Phase 1

United States
Utah Locations

Salt Lake City, Utah, United States, 84132
Moran Eye Center, University of Utah

Eligibility Criteria
Description

Inclusion Criteria
- All nonpregnant, nonlactating adults with normal vision in both eyes

Exclusion Criteria
- Previous ocular pathologies

Ages Eligible for Study
18–65 Years (Adult, Older Adult)

Sexes Eligible for Study
All

Accepts Healthy Volunteers
Yes
Study Plan

Design Details
Primary Purpose: Treatment
Allocation: Randomized
Interventional Model: Parallel Assignment
Masking: Triple (Participant Investigator Outcomes Assessor)

Arms and interventions

Participant group/arm	Intervention/treatment
Experimental: 1	Drug: 4-Methylpyrazole • 15 mg/kg dose
Placebo Comparator: 2 Saline	Other: saline

Primary outcome measures

Outcome measure	Measure description	Time frame
Dark adaptation inhibition measured 30 min after drug infusion using Goldman-Weeker adaptometer.		6 weeks

Sponsor
University of Utah

Collaborators
No information provided

Investigators
• Principal Investigator: Paul S Bernstein, M.D., Ph.D., University of Utah

General Publications
No publications available

United States

Completed

**Effect of DHA Supplements on Macular Function in Patients
with Stargardt Macular Dystrophy and Stargardt-like Macular Dystrophy**

ClinicalTrials.gov ID NCT00060749

Sponsor National Eye Institute (NEI)
Information provided by National Institutes of Health Clinical Center (CC)
Last Update Posted 2017-07-02

Study Overview

Brief Summary

This study will evaluate whether docosahexaenoic acid (DHA) dietary supplementation can improve macular function in patients with Stargardt macular dystrophy and Stargardt-like macular dystrophy. Stargardt macular dystrophy is a recessive inherited trait that causes a severe form of macular degeneration. (The macula is the center part of the retina in the back of the eye that is responsible for fine vision.) The disorder begins in late childhood and progresses to a significant decrease in central vision. One of the earliest signs of the disorder is accumulation in and under the macula of a fatty pigment called lipofuscin. Stargardt-like macular dystrophy is a dominant inherited trait involving loss of central vision, but it begins later than Stargardt macular dystrophy, and the accumulation of lipofuscin extends beyond the central region of the macula. DHA is a fatty acid that is essential for normal brain and eye development. It is normally found in the diet, but not in large amounts. Supplements may help prevent or slow the progression of some eye diseases.

Patients with autosomal dominant Stargardt-like macular dystrophy or autosomal recessive Stargardt macular dystrophy are eligible for this study. Candidates will be screened with the following tests and procedures:

- Medical history and physical examination.
- Blood test to measure levels of DHA and vitamins.
- Eye examination: The patient's vision and eye pressure are tested, then the pupils are dilated to examine structures inside the eye. Photographs are also taken.
- Visual field test: The patient looks at a tiny spot of light projected onto a white screen and is asked to note when other lights appear at other places on the screen.
- Electroretinogram (ERG): An electrode (small silver disk) is taped to the patient's forehead. Drops are given to numb the eyes and special contact lenses are inserted in the eyes. For the first part of the test, the patient looks at the center of a black and white checkerboard screen that flickers for 30 s at a time. This is repeated 16 or more times. For the second part of the test, the patient looks inside a sphere, in which flashes of light flicker for 20 s at a time. This is repeated four or more times. The contact lenses sense small electrical signals generated by the retina during the tests.

Participants will begin taking DHA capsules or a placebo (look-alike capsules with no active ingredient) from 1 week to 3 months after enrolling in the study and will repeat several of the screening tests at follow-up visits scheduled 3, 6, 9, 12, and 15 months after they start taking the capsules. They will also be interviewed about any treatment side effects.

Detailed Description

We propose to undertake a double-masked, randomized, placebo-controlled, crossover study on the effect of docosahexaenoic acid (DHA) dietary supplementation in subjects with macular dystrophy to determine whether DHA can improve macular function. Subjects will receive either oral DHA supplementation (5×200 mg BID, 2,000 mg/day) or placebo. Subjects will 'crossover' to the opposite treatment twice during this study. Primary outcomes will measure the change in macular function during periods with and without DHA supplementation.

Zhang and colleagues found a mutation in the gene, ELOVL4 (elongation of the very long chain fatty acid-4), in individuals with Stargardt-like macular dystrophy. The gene is presumed to function in the pathway of synthesis of very long chain polyunsaturated fatty acids, including DHA. DHA is the major very long chain polyunsaturated fatty acid of the retina. As our North American diet is poor in DHA, we hypothesize that a DHA dietary supplement might improve macular function in individuals with the ELOVL4 mutation. Since the effect of DHA supplementation may be nonspecific, we propose to study a second cohort with Stargardt macular dystrophy, which has a different genotype involving a different metabolic pathway in the eye, but presents with a similar phenotype. Two cohorts of up to 10 subjects for analysis will be recruited from patients with either Stargardt-like macular dystrophy or Stargardt macular dystrophy.

Official Title

Investigation of the Effect of Dietary Docosahexaenoic Acid (DHA) Supplementation on Macular Function in Subjects with Autosomal Dominant Stargardt-Like and Autosomal Recessive Stargardt Macular Dystrophy

Conditions

Macular Degeneration

Intervention/Treatment

- Drug: Docosahexaenoic Acid (DHA) Dietary Supplement

Other Study ID Numbers

- 030179
- 03-EI-0179

Study Start

2003-05-05

Primary Completion

Study Completion
2007-12-10

Enrollment

22

Study Type

Interventional

Phase

Phase 1

United States
Maryland Locations

Bethesda, Maryland, United States, 20892
National Institutes of Health Clinical Center, 9000 Rockville Pike

Eligibility Criteria
Description

Inclusion Criteria
To be eligible to enroll in this study, a prospective participant must satisfy the following inclusion criteria.

- Understand and sign the informed consent.
- Able to comply with all study procedures (likely to exclude participants less than 10 years of age, but not necessarily).

Autosomal Recessive Stargardt Macular Dystrophy Participants (must be observed in at least one study eye):

- Have a pattern of inheritance that indicates autosomal recessive inheritance.
- Have a phenotype consistent with the diagnosis of autosomal recessive Stargardt macular dystrophy including the following clinical features: fundus examination showing bilateral central maculopathy and/or fundus flecks, or characteristic changes on an intravenous fluorescein angiogram.

Autosomal Dominant Stargardt-like Macular Dystrophy Participants (must be observed in at least one study eye):

- Have a pattern of inheritance that indicates autosomal dominant inheritance.
- Have a phenotype consistent with the diagnosis of Stargardt-like macular dystrophy that may include: fundus examination showing bilateral central maculopathy and fundus flecks confined to the central macula, or intravenous fluorescein angiogram.

Exclusion Criteria
To be eligible to enroll in this study, a prospective participant must not satisfy any of the following exclusion criteria.

- Have a non-recordable multifocal ERG.

Ages Eligible for Study
(Child, Adult, Older Adult)

Sexes Eligible for Study
All

Accepts Healthy Volunteers
No
Study Plan

Design Details
Primary Purpose: Treatment

Arms and interventions

Intervention/treatment
Drug: Docosahexaenoic Acid (DHA) Dietary Supplement

Sponsor
National Eye Institute (NEI)

Collaborators
No information provided

Investigators
No information provided

General Publications
- Zhang K, Kniazeva M, Han M, Li W, Yu Z, Yang Z, Li Y, Metzker ML, Allikmets R, Zack DJ, Kakuk LE, Lagali PS, Wong PW, MacDonald IM, Sieving PA, Figueroa DJ, Austin CP, Gould RJ, Ayyagari R, Petrukhin K. A 5-bp deletion in ELOVL4 is associated with two related forms of autosomal dominant macular dystrophy. Nat Genet. 2001 Jan;27(1):89–93. https://doi.org/10.1038/83817.

United States

Completed

Long-Term Follow-Up of Subretinal Transplantation of hESC-Derived RPE Cells in Stargardt Macular Dystrophy Patients

ClinicalTrials.gov ID NCT02445612

Sponsor Astellas Institute for Regenerative Medicine
Information provided by Astellas Pharma Inc (Astellas Institute for Regenerative Medicine) (Responsible Party)
Last Update Posted 2020-11-13

Study Overview

Brief Summary
The purpose of this study is to evaluate the long-term safety and tolerability of MA09-hRPE cellular therapy in patients with advanced Stargardt's Macular Dystrophy (SMD) from 1 to 5 years following the surgical procedure to implant the MA09-hRPE cells.

Detailed Description
This study is a long-term, follow-up to the ACT MA09-hRPE 001 phase I/II trial; the phase I/II trial (referred to as the core protocol) was an open-label, non-randomized, dose escalation, multicenter trial. Thirteen SMD patients were treated in this trial. Ten patients with profound vision loss (visual acuity <=20/400) received a single subretinal injection of MA09-hRPE cells, starting at a dose of 50,000 MA09-hRPE cells (three patients), 100,000 MA09-hRPE cells transplanted (three patients), 150,000 MA09-hRPE cells transplanted (three patients), and increasing to

a maximum dose of 200,000 MA09-hRPE cells transplanted (one patient). Three patients with severe to moderate vision loss (visual acuity <= 20/100) received a dose of 100,000 MA09-hRPE cells. All patients who participated in the core protocol are eligible for participation in this follow-up protocol.

The first visit of this long-term follow-up protocol will correspond to the last visit of the core protocol and will take place at 12 months post-cell implantation. Informed consent will be obtained at this visit.

Patients will be evaluated at 18, 24, 36, 48, and 60 months posttransplant (or more frequently as clinically indicated). Follow-up will include obtaining information about ophthalmological findings and events of special interest as defined in the Primary Outcomes. At the last visit of this follow-up study, whether at 60 months posttransplant or at early discontinuation, patients will be invited to participate in a Safety Surveillance Study for an additional 10 years, under a separate protocol, which will continue to monitor the long-term risks of MA09-hRPE cell transplantation.

Official Title

Long-Term Follow-Up to a Phase I/II, Open-Label, Multicenter, Prospective Study to Determine the Safety and Tolerability of Subretinal Transplantation of Human Embryonic Stem Cell-Derived Retinal Pigmented Epithelial (MA09-hRPE) Cells in Patients With Stargardt's Macular Dystrophy (SMD)

Conditions

Stargardt's Macular Dystrophy

Intervention/Treatment

- Biological: MA09-hRPE

Other Study ID Numbers

- 7316-CL-0004
- ACT MA09-hRPE 001(SMD)LTFU (Other Identifier) (OTHER: Sponsor)

Study Start (Actual)

2012-07-11

Primary Completion (Actual)

2019-06-21

Study Completion (Actual)

2019-06-21

Enrollment (Actual)

13

Study Type

Observational

United States
California Locations

Los Angeles, California, United States, 90095
Jules Stein Eye Institute, UCLA School of Medicine

Florida Locations

Miami, Florida, United States, 33136
Bascom Palmer Eye Institute

Pennsylvania Locations

Philadelphia, Pennsylvania, United States, 19107
Wills Eye Institute-Mid Atlantic Retina

Description

Inclusion Criteria
- Must have been treated with hESC-RPE cell transplant in the core protocol.
- Able to understand and willing to sign the informed consent to participate in the follow-up study.

Exclusion Criteria
- There are no exclusion criteria

Study Population
The study population is by invitation only for previous participants in the core protocol.

Ages Eligible for Study
18 Years and older (Adult, Older Adult)

Sexes Eligible for Study
All

Accepts Healthy Volunteers
No
Sampling Method
Non-Probability Sample

Design Details
Observational Model: Cohort
Time Perspective: Prospective

Cohorts and interventions

Group/cohort	Intervention/treatment
Experimental: MA09-hRPE Subretinal transplantation of MA09-hRPE cells	Biological: MA09-hRPE • Cohort 1 50,000 cells Cohort 2 100,000 cells Cohort 2a Better Vision 100,000 cells Cohort 3 150,000 cells Cohort 4 200,000 cells • Other Names: – ASP7316

Primary outcome measures

Outcome measure	Measure description	Time frame
Safety assessed by Adverse Events (AEs) of special interest in regard to the investigational product	This will include obtaining information about ophthalmological findings and Serious Adverse Events (SAEs) that are neurologic, infectious, hematologic, or fatal, pregnancy in a female subject or the partner of a male subject and pregnancy outcome, any adverse event (AE) that causes a subject to withdraw from the study, any new diagnosis of an ocular or immune-mediated disorder, cancer, ectopic or proliferative cell growth (Retinal pigment epithelium (RPE) or non-RPE) with adverse clinical consequence, and unexpected, clinically significant AEs possibly related to the cell transplant procedure or the investigational product (MA09-hRPE cells).	4 years

Secondary outcome measures

Outcome measure	Measure description	Time frame
Incidence of graft failure or rejection	Evidence of graft failure or rejection will consist of: Presence of retinal edema, cystoid macular edema, retinal white dots, retinal hemorrhage, serous retinal detachment, subretinal exudates, subretinal fibrosis, or vascular and/or optic disc leakage, elevated intraocular pressure or hypotony. Evidence of unanticipated and persistent or increasing noninfectious ocular inflammation (e.g., vasculitis, retinitis, choroiditis, vitritis, pars planitis, anterior segment inflammation/uveitis).	4 years
Number of patients with changes in ocular examinations or images	The number of patients with clinically significant absolute values or changes from baseline in Intraocular pressure (IOP) and Best-Corrected Visual Acuity (BCVA) will be summarized.	4 years

Sponsor
Astellas Institute for Regenerative Medicine

Collaborators
No information provided

Investigators
• Study Director: Medical Director, Astellas Institute for Regenerative Medicine

General Publications
No publications available

United States

Completed

Subretinal Transplantation of hESC-Derived RPE(MA09-hRPE)Cells in Patients with Stargardt's Macular Dystrophy

ClinicalTrials.gov ID NCT01345006

Sponsor Astellas Institute for Regenerative Medicine
Information provided by Astellas Pharma Inc (Astellas Institute for Regenerative Medicine) (Responsible Party)
Last Update Posted 2021-07-07

Study Overview

Brief Summary
This is a safety and tolerability trial to evaluate the effect of subretinal injection of human embryonic stem cell-derived retinal pigment epithelium cells in patients with Stargardt's Macular Dystrophy (SMD).

Detailed Description
This study is a Phase I/II, open-label, non-randomized, sequential, multicenter clinical trial. There will be 5 cohorts, the 4 low vision cohorts will contain 3 patients, the better vision cohort will contain 4 patients.

The enrolled cohorts will be as follows:

Three SMD patients- 50,000 MA09-hRPE cells transplanted
Three SMD patients- 100,000 MA09-hRPE cells transplanted
Four Better Vison SMD patients- 100,000 MA09-hRPE cells transplanted
Three SMD patients- 150,000 MA09-hRPE cells transplanted
Three SMD patients- 200,000 MA09-hRPE cells transplanted

Patients will be enrolled sequentially, and within each cohort of 3 patients, each patient's clinical course over the first 6 weeks following cell transplantation will be reviewed by an independent DSMB before enrollment is opened for the next 2 patients. A full safety assessment of all 3 patients in each cohort will be made by the DSMB when the 3rd patient in each cohort completes 4 weeks of follow-up, and before the first patient in the next cohort receives a cell transplant. The exception is the better vision group where all patients may be enrolled once DSMB approval has been received.

Each cohort will be enrolled sequentially in turn, with the exception of the better vision cohort which may be enrolled in parallel with the other cohorts.

The day of the cell implantation will be Day 0, and patients will remain in the study until the last visit at 12 months.

Official Title
A Phase I/II, Open-Label, Multicenter, Prospective Study to Determine the Safety
and Tolerability of Subretinal Transplantation of Human Embryonic Stem Cell-
Derived Retinal Pigmented Epithelial (MA09-hRPE) Cells in Patients With
Stargardt's Macular Dystrophy (SMD)

Conditions
Stargardt's Macular Dystrophy

Intervention/Treatment
- Biological: MA09-hRPE

Other Study ID Numbers
- 7316-CL-0001
- ACT SMD 01 MA09-hRPE (Other Identifier) (OTHER: Sponsor)
- ACT MA09-hRPE SMD-001 (Other Identifier) (OTHER: Sponsor)

Study Start (Actual)
2011-06-16

Primary Completion (Actual)
2015-08-10

Study Completion (Actual)
2015-08-10

Enrollment (Actual)
13

Study Type
Interventional

Phase
Phase 1 and Phase 2

United States
California Locations

Los Angeles, California, United States, 90095
Jules Stein Eye Institute, UCLA School of Medicine

Florida Locations

Miami, Florida, United States, 33136
Bascom Palmer Eye institute

Pennsylvania Locations

Philadelphia, Pennsylvania, United States, 19107
Wills Eye Institute-Mid Atlantic Retina

Eligibility Criteria
Description

Inclusion Criteria
- Adult male or female over 18 years of age.
- Clinical diagnosis of advanced SMD.
- If known, the patient's genotype will be recorded in the medical history; if unknown, patient will allow for the submission of a sample for genotyping. Clinical findings consistent with SMD.
- The visual acuity of the eye to receive the transplant will be no better than 20/400. The visual acuity of the eye in the better vision cohort to receive the transplant will be no better than 20/100.
- The visual acuity of the eye that is not to receive the transplant will be no better than 20/400 for the worse vision patients and no worse than 20/100 for the better vision patients.
- Peripheral visual field constriction documented on standard kinetic visual field testing.
- Electrophysiological findings consistent with SMD.
- Medically suitable to undergo vitrectomy and subretinal injection.
- Medically suitable for general anesthesia or waking sedation, if needed.
- Medically suitable for transplantation of an embryonic stem cell line:
- Normal serum chemistry (sequential multichannel analyzer 20 [SMA- 20]) and hematology (complete blood count [CBC], prothrombin time [PT], and activated partial thromboplastin time [aPTT]) screening tests.
- Negative urine screen for drugs of abuse.
- Negative human immunodeficiency virus (HIV), hepatitis B (HBV), hepatitis C (HCV) serologies.
- No history of malignancy, with the exception of successfully treated basal cell or squamous cell carcinoma of the skin.
- Negative cancer screening within previous 6 months:
- Complete history and physical examination;
- Dermatological screening exam for malignant lesions;
- Negative fecal occult blood test and if over age 50 years, negative colonoscopy within previous 7 years;
- Negative chest roentgenogram (CXR);
- Normal CBC and manual differential;
- Negative urinalysis (U/A);
- Normal thyroid exam;
- If male, normal testicular examination; if over age 40, digital rectal examination (DRE) and prostate-specific antigen (PSA);
- If female, normal pelvic examination with Papanicolaou smear; and
- If female, normal clinical breast exam and if 40 years of age or older, negative mammogram.
- If female and of childbearing potential, willing to use two effective forms of birth control during the study.
- If male, willing to use barrier and spermicide contraception during the study.
- Willing to defer all future blood, blood component, or tissue donation. -Able to understand and willing to sign the informed consent.

Exclusion Criteria

- History of malignancy, with the exception of successfully treated basal cell or squamous cell carcinoma of the skin.
- History of myocardial infarction in previous 12 months.
- History of diabetes mellitus.
- Any immunodeficiency.
- Any current immunosuppressive therapy other than intermittent or low-dose corticosteroids.
- Serologic evidence of infection with Hepatitis B, Hepatitis C, or HIV.
- Current participation in any other clinical trial.
- Participation within previous 6 months in any clinical trial of a drug by ocular or systemic administration.
- Any other sight-threatening ocular disease.
- Any chronic ocular medications.
- Any history of retinal vascular disease (compromised blood-retinal barrier.
- Glaucoma.
- Uveitis or other intraocular inflammatory disease.
- Significant lens opacities or other media opacity.
- Ocular lens removal within previous 3 months.
- If female, pregnancy or lactation.
- Any other medical condition, which, in the investigator's judgment, will interfere with the patient's ability to comply with the protocol, compromises patient safety, or interferes with the interpretation of the study results.

Ages Eligible for Study

18 Years and older (Adult, Older Adult)

Sexes Eligible for Study

All

Accepts Healthy Volunteers

No

Design Details

Primary Purpose: Other
Allocation: N/A
Interventional Model: Single Group Assignment
Masking: None (Open Label)

Arms and interventions

Participant group/arm	Intervention/treatment
Experimental: MA09-hRPE Patients will undergo subretinal injection of MA09-hRPE	Biological: MA09-hRPE • Cohort 1 50,000 cells Cohort 2 100,000 cells Cohort 2a Better Vision 100,000 cells Cohort 3 150,000 cells Cohort 4 200,000 cells

Primary outcome measures

Outcome measure	Measure description	Time frame
The safety and tolerance of transplantation of hESC-derived RPE cells MA09-hRPE	The transplantation of hESC-derived RPE cells MA09-hRPE will be considered safe and tolerated in the absence of: • Any grade 2 (NCI grading system) or greater adverse event related to the cell product • Any evidence that the cells are contaminated with an infectious agent • Any evidence that the cells show tumorigenic potential	12 months
Safety Assessments	• Adverse Event and Serious Adverse Event assessment • Clinical monitoring • Serial vital signs • Clinical laboratory tests • Directed ophthalmological monitoring • Monitoring of RPE cells' acceptance/integrity/rejection • Monitoring of local and systemic infection • Monitoring of tumorigenic cell transformation	12 months

Secondary outcome measures

Outcome measure	Measure description	Time frame
Evidence of successful engraftment	Evidence of successful engraftment will consist of: • Structural evidence (OCT imaging, fluorescein angiography, autofluorescence photography, slit-lamp examination with fundus photography) that cells have been implanted in the correct location • Electroretinographic evidence (mfERG) showing enhanced activity in the implant location	12 months

Sponsor
Astellas Institute for Regenerative Medicine

Collaborators
No information provided

Investigators
• Study Director: Medical Director, Astellas Institute for Regenerative Medicine

General Publications
No publications available

Brazil

Completed

Stem Cell Therapy for Outer Retinal Degenerations

ClinicalTrials.gov ID NCT02903576

Sponsor Federal University of São Paulo
Information provided by Rubens Belfort Jr., Federal University of São Paulo
  (Responsible Party)
Last Update Posted 2020-07-22

Study Overview

Brief Summary

This study is a Phase I/II, open-label, non-randomized, prospective study to determine the safety of human embryonic stem cell-derived retinal pigmented epithelium (hESC RPE) subretinal injections versus hESC RPE seeded on a polymeric substrate implanted in the subretinal space.

Detailed Description

To determine whether the surgical implantation of a human embryonic stem cell-derived retinal pigmented epithelium (hESC-RPE) monolayer seeded onto a polymeric versus hESC-RPE injections into the subretinal space is a safe procedure.

Six patients will receive hESC-RPE cell injections (100000 cells) in the subretinal space (2 Dry Age-related macular degeneration (AMD), 2 Wet AMD with disciform scar, and 2 with Stargardt's disease).

Also, 5 patients with Dry AMD, 5 patients with Wet AMD with disciform scar, and 5 patients with Stargardt's disease will receive a subretinal implantation of the hESC-RPE seeded in a monolayer in a polymeric substrate.

Patients will be enrolled sequentially, and after the procedure, the patients will be followed for 1 year.

Official Title

Stem Cell-Derived Retinal Pigmented Epithelium Implantation in Patients With Outer Retinal Degenerations: Phase I/II Clinical Trial

Conditions

Age-Related Macular Degeneration
Stargardt's Disease
Exudative Age-related Macular Degeneration

Intervention/Treatment

- Procedure: injection of hESC-RPE in suspension
- Procedure: injection hESC-RPE seeded in a substrate

Other Study ID Numbers
- 12018712.5.0000.5505

Study Start
2015-08

Primary Completion (Actual)
2019-01

Study Completion (Actual)
2019-06

Enrollment (Actual)
15

Study Type
Interventional

Phase
Phase 1 and Phase 2

Brazil

Sao Paulo, Brazil, 04023-062
Federal University of Sao Paulo

Eligibility Criteria
Description

Inclusion Criteria
- Patients with AMD (Dry, Wet after failure of treatment, disciform scars)
- Patients with Stargardt's Disease BCVA on the selected eye: worse than 20/200

Exclusion Criteria
- Other ophthalmological diseases (Glaucoma, Diabetic Retinopathy, Previous retinal surgery, uveitis)
- Systemic diseases with contraindication for surgical procedures with local anesthesia

Ages Eligible for Study
18–90 Years (Adult, Older Adult)

Sexes Eligible for Study
All

Accepts Healthy Volunteers
No

Design Details
Primary Purpose: Treatment
Allocation: Non-Randomized
Interventional Model: Parallel Assignment
Masking: None (Open Label)

Arms and interventions

Participant group/arm	Intervention/treatment
Active Comparator: injection of hESC-RPE in suspension 6 patients will receive cell suspension injections on the subretinal space prior to the surgeries, to access safety	Procedure: injection of hESC-RPE in suspension • The first six patients will receive a subretinal injection of hESC-RPE in solution after a complete pars plana vitrectomy to access safety of the cell implant alone. • Other Names: – Human Embryonic Stem Cell—Retinal Pigmented Epithelium
Active Comparator: injection hESC-RPE seeded in a substrate 15 patients will receive a subretinal implantation of a polymeric scaffold seeded hESC-RPE in monolayer	Procedure: injection hESC-RPE seeded in a substrate • Fifteen patients will receive a subretinal implantation of embryonic stem cell-derived retinal pigmented epithelium seeded in a polymeric substrate to access safety of substrate seeded with RPE • Other Names: – Human Embryonic Stem Cell seeded in a polymeric substrate

Primary outcome measures

Outcome measure	Measure description	Time frame
Incidence of treatment-emergent adverse events of subretinal implantation of stem cell-derived retinal pigmented epithelium in the subretinal space.	Incidence of surgical-related side effects: retinal detachment, ocular inflammation, increase in intraocular pressure, infection (endophthalmitis), loss of vision due to surgical-related complications	1 year

Secondary outcome measures

Outcome measure	Measure description	Time frame
Incidence of side effects related to the treatment itself (injection and implantation of subretinal stem cell-related RPE)	Inflammation/rejection cell migration/ differentiation tumor formation proliferative vitreoretinopathy/retinal detachment implant migration	1 year

Sponsor
Federal University of São Paulo

Collaborators
No information provided

Investigators
• Study Chair: Rubens Belfort, MD, Federal University of São Paulo UNIFESP

General Publications
No publications available

China

Completed

The Effect of Duration Between Sessions on Microperimetric Biofeedback Training in Patients with Maculopathies

ClinicalTrials.gov ID NCT05904444

Sponsor Aier Eye Hospital, Guangzhou
Information provided by Jie Zhou, Aier Eye Hospital, Guangzhou (Responsible Party)
Last Update Posted 2023-06-15

Study Overview

Brief Summary

Patients who develop macular diseases have several clinical complications, such as central vision loss, the central scotoma of the visual field, the decrease of reading speed, and fixation stability. At present, there is still no satisfactory effect in the prevention and treatment of advanced macular disease. A new rehabilitation strategy named microperimetric biofeedback training has been shown to be effective in improving patients' visual appearance, but there is no consensus regarding the optimal methodology and standard of practice. Therefore, we designed a prospective clinical study to verify the effectiveness of MBFT and to determine an optimal plan.

Detailed Description

The present study aimed to investigate the effects of training frequency and number of training sessions on the visual outcomes of patients with various macular diseases. A total of 15 training sessions were conducted on two distinct frequencies, namely once a day and once every other day. Baseline measurements included fixation stability, reading speed, and best-corrected visual acuity (BCVA) which were obtained and followed up after the 5, 10, and 15 training sessions. By comparing the changes in these visual function parameters across different stages of training, the study aimed to identify and analyze the underlying patterns and rules governing the training process. Ultimately, the results of this study could serve as a valuable reference for standardizing the use of MBFT in clinical practice.

Official Title

The Effect of Duration Between Sessions on Microperimetric Biofeedback Training in Patients with Maculopathies

Conditions

Macular Degeneration
Low Vision
Stargardt Disease

Intervention/Treatment
- Procedure: microperimetric biofeedback training

Other Study ID Numbers
- GZAIER2018IRB11

Study Start (Actual)
2018-08-15

Primary Completion (Actual)
2023-04-30

Study Completion (Actual)
2023-04-30

Enrollment (Actual)
29

Study Type
Interventional

Phase
Not Applicable

China
Guangdong Locations

Guangzhou, Guangdong, China, 510000
MAIA microperimetry

Eligibility Criteria
Description

Inclusion Criteria
Participants who:

- were diagnosed with macular disease and had a BCVA poorer than 20/60;
- with stable fundus lesion in fundus examinations;
- with education level beyond the third grade;
- had no other effective treatment; and
- were willing to improve visual quality.

Exclusion Criteria
who:

- received ocular treatments in the preceding 3 months,
- with active fundus lesions like inflammation, bleeding, exudation, and edema,
- with obvious opacity of the refractive media such as keratopathy, severe cataract, or severe vitreous opacity,
- were unable to attend scheduled follow-up appointments.

Ages Eligible for Study
12–80 Years (Child, Adult, Older Adult)

Sexes Eligible for Study
All

Accepts Healthy Volunteers
No
Study Plan

Design Details
Primary Purpose: Treatment
Allocation: Non-Randomized
Interventional Model: Single Group Assignment
Masking: None (Open Label)

Arms and interventions

Participant group/arm	Intervention/treatment
Experimental: daily training Patients underwent microperimetric training everyday	Procedure: microperimetric biofeedback training • Microperimetry biofeedback training is a noninvasive strategy to develop a new trained retinal locus or strengthen the spontaneous preferred retinal locus to get better visual performances. The rationale of MBFT consists of reeducating visual system to a new visual condition, promoting retina-brain transmission, and further enhancing synaptic plasticity and neural capacity by acoustic biofeedback or structured light stimulus biofeedback.
Experimental: alternately training Patients underwent microperimetric training every other day	Procedure: microperimetric biofeedback training • Microperimetry biofeedback training is a noninvasive strategy to develop a new trained retinal locus or strengthen the spontaneous preferred retinal locus to get better visual performance. The rationale of MBFT consists of reeducating visual system to a new visual condition, promoting retina-brain transmission, and further enhancing synaptic plasticity and neural capacity by acoustic biofeedback or structured light stimulus biofeedback.

Primary outcome measures

Outcome measure	Measure description	Time frame
Fixation stability	An index for evaluating macular disease, defined as the accuracy of a patient's gaze at a target over a period of time.	5 min

Secondary outcome measures

Outcome measure	Measure description	Time frame
Best-corrected visual acuity	The most important indicator of visual function refers to the function of distinguishing objects in the state of refractive correction.	2 min

Outcome measure	Measure description	Time frame
Reading speed	One of the indicators for evaluating reading ability, which refers to the number of words within a certain period of time when reading	3 min
Questionnaires	Questionnaires were used to determine the influence of eye symptoms and visual impairment on daily life attributed to the limitation of patients' social function and activities.	10 min

Sponsor
Aier Eye Hospital, Guangzhou

Collaborators
No information provided

Investigators
- Study Director: Jinling Zhang, Doctor, Aier Eye Hospital, Guangzhou

General Publications
No publications available

Columbia

Completed

Efficacy of Acupuncture in Macular Diseases (AMAD)

ClinicalTrials.gov ID NCT02255981

Sponsor Escuela Neijing
Information provided by Dra. Luz Helena Gutiérrez C, Escuela Neijing (Responsible Party)
Last Update Posted 2020-06-16

Study Overview

Brief Summary
This is a single-arm study designed to assess the efficacy of acupuncture (Traditional Chinese Medicine) for chronic macular diseases of several types. All participants received acupuncture and massage and there is no placebo group because it is not considered a good form to evaluate in Chinese Medicine due to, acupuncturing being a procedure is not as blind as is desired. As a control of the results in this trial, the outcomes could be contrasted against those reported in known medical publications and against expectations of the progress of the damage without treatment.

Detailed Description

Background

WHO has included retinal diseases between conditions treatable by acupuncture and Traditional Chinese Medicine (TCM) has been used for retinal diseases in hospitals of China and in other parts of the world many years ago. Acupuncture and periocular massage act stimulating the vital energy to restore the normal function of the body.

Currently, most common treatments in Western Medicine, anti-VEGF, only are indicated for less than 10% of cases, which are the wet form or neovascular of AMD (NV-AMD) and they have restrictions for use; additionally, their cost and requirements are limiting for populations in all countries.

Objectives. The primary purpose of this study is to confirm the objective response among subjects with macular diseases treated with acupuncture and massage. The results of conventional treatment are published in similar trials and some of our patients have had intraocular injections previously.

It is important to feature the affordability of this therapy for low-income populations who do not have specialists or facilities nearby or for many governments that complain about the huge burden of the treatment of their diseases. In Colombia, the average cost of each intraocular injection by the time of this trial was about US 3.500 and it can be repeated every month; it requires a retina specialist and a surgical room which are out of reach for many people in the country.

We did not calculate the costs of our treatment because the research team did voluntary labor, and the devices are at a very low cost, about US 0.50 in each session. Acupuncture treatment does not require special facilities as surgical rooms required in treatments with intraocular injections. The participants were not paid; they came from different economic conditions, some better, others from poorest neighborhoods or some from the rural areas.

This study includes 3 phases: Selection, Treatment, and Follow-up phases.

The selection phase included confirmed diagnosis by clinical register and OCT, ophthalmologic assessment, and consent of the patient.

Macular diseases. In this trial, some patients had NV AMD in one or both eyes, dry AMD, myopic maculopathy, or Stargardt disease. For TCM, it is possible to treat all as damage of similar category.

Why no control group? There was no control group due to ethical reasons; leave the impairment without treatment in these mostly very sad persons. The second reason is the well-known difficulty to mask a procedure like acupuncture. The third reason is the possibility to contrast the results of this trial with those of similar studies conducted in eyes with conventional treatment.

In the phase of treatment, patients received a session of acupuncture according to a standard protocol of points and a periocular massage that was taught to the patient to be self-performed daily. The acupuncture sessions were scheduled every week initially; the evaluation of response was realized every 2 months by ophthalmologic exam. Participants performed optical coherence tomography (OCT) every 6 months.

Depending on the results of ophthalmologic assessment, the sessions were extended gradually to every 2, 3, 5, until 13 weeks. Although tomographic assessments had been scheduled every 6 months, only a few of the participants accomplish that due to economic limitations. Treatment continued until 24 months.

All patients in the follow-up phase of this trial were monitored according to the Safety Follow-up protocol and the defined procedures and evaluations.

The final results were collected and analyzed.

Official Title
¿Es Util la Acupuntura en la Degeneracion Macular? Prospective Study of Efficacy of Acupuncture in Macular Diseases

Conditions
Age-related Macular Degeneration
Stargardt Disease
Macular Dystrophy

Intervention/Treatment
• Other: Acupuncture and massage

Other Study ID Numbers
• Neijing Ophthalmology

Study Start
2013-03

Primary Completion (Actual)
2016-05

Study Completion (Actual)
2016-11

Enrollment (Actual)
33

Study Type
Interventional

Phase
Not Applicable

Colombia
Antioquia Locations

Guarne, Antioquia, Colombia, 0000
IPS Fundación Neijing

Medellin, Antioquia, Colombia, 0000
IPS Fundación Neijing

Eligibility Criteria
Description

Inclusion Criteria
- Clinical diagnosis of Macular Disease.

  - The patient must accept treatment with acupuncture

Exclusion Criteria
- None

Ages Eligible for Study
(Child, Adult, Older Adult)

Sexes Eligible for Study
All

Accepts Healthy Volunteers
No

Design Details
Primary Purpose: Treatment
Allocation: N/A
Interventional Model: Single Group Assignment
Interventional Model Description: Interventional, no randomized, no masking
Masking: None (Open Label)
Masking Description: Masking is neither accurate nor reliable in a procedure such
    as acupuncture or massage.

Arms and interventions

Participant group/arm	Intervention/treatment

Experimental: Acupuncture group
Acupuncture and massage therapy of traditional Chinese medicine (acupuncture and massage) for 24 months
	Other: Acupuncture and massage
	• Treatment consists of putting needles on specific points of skin one day each week initially, then with longer spaces of time according to improvement. A total of 11 Chinese needles of stainless steel, 25 × 40, were used by manual insertion and left for 12–15 min.
	Periocular massage is taught and is practiced daily by the patient himself or herself.
	• Other Names:
	  – Traditional Chinese Medicine: (TCM)
	  – Acupuncture Chinese style

Primary outcome measures

Outcome measure	Measure description	Time frame
Change on visual acuity (VA) of the treated eyes from baseline to the end of the study	The primary objective is to assess if acupuncture treatment is linked to a change in visual acuity (VA). VA was obtained by an ophthalmologic assessment at baseline and every two months until month 24. VA measurements were taken with the patient in a sitting position using a Snellen chart at a testing distance of 6 meters. The scale in Snellen is given in fractional numbers corresponding 20/20 to a normal vision at 20 ft or 6 meters. According to the World Health Organization, the normal vision is to 20/25, severe impairment corresponds to VA worse than 20/200 or legal blindness. Each fraction corresponds to a determined line of the chart in which all letters are correctly identified and the variation or gain is appreciated by the lines gained or lost by each eye. Improvement means a fraction better than initial, stable is no change in VA, and lost is the VA worse than that of baseline.	Baseline, 2 months and every 2 months until month 24.
Eyes with change from baseline to the end of the study in distance vision according to categories CIE 10 based on lines seen on the Snellen Chart.	Change in visual acuity was measured by the number of lines seen on the Snellen Chart from baseline to the end of the trial. The measure was obtained by an ophthalmologic assessment on both eyes at the beginning of the study and every two months until month 24 using the best correction. VA measurements (lines in which all letters are correctly identified) were performed with the patient in a sitting position using a Snellen chart at a testing distance of 6 meters and the variation is appreciated by the lines gained or lost by each eye. The measure in Snellen is given in fractional numbers. Each fraction corresponds to a determined line of the chart corresponding VA 20/20 or 6/6 to a normal vision at 20 ft or 6 meters. The range of normal vision according to the WHO is to 20/25 ft or 6/10m, Mild means VA worse than 6/12, Moderate means VA worse than 6/18, Severe means VA worse than 6/60 that is "legal blindness". Blindness is considered VA worse than 3/60.	24 months from baseline.
Change from baseline in the number of letters seen on the Early-Treatment Diabetic Retinopathy Study (ETDRS) Eye Chart	The ETDRS scale of letters is commonly used to report outcomes in AMD; for this reason, this score was chosen to compare outcomes with similar studies. Accepted tables for conversion from Snellen to ETDRS were used. Eighty-five letters are equivalent to 20/20 and 0 letters correspond to 20/200. It can be meaningful to analyze the results in this trial in the context of similar trials using anti-VEGF, or reporting a visual loss in those cases that are not treatable.	Baseline and at end of study (up to 2 years)

Outcome measure	Measure description	Time frame
Number of eyes that improved VA from baseline to end of the study in participants with different forms of macular disease treated with acupuncture.	"Improved" was defined as cases that gained in visual acuity (Note: no minimum of letters was defined). "Stable" was defined as visual acuity that did not change in the sense of not losing or gaining in the final identification of the optotypes. "Lost" was defined as patients who had a worse vision at the end than at the beginning (e.g., lost visual acuity because the disease continued its course and the treatment was not effective.)	2 years

Secondary outcome measures

Outcome measure	Measure description	Time frame
Percentage of participants who experienced changes in vision (Less opacity, less distortion of lines, reduction of the central shadow)	At study entry, major complaints of patients were collected by survey. Participants also completed a survey at the middle and at the end of the trial. These data are the percentage of participants who reported changes to the main visual complaints that they considered significant in their lives compared with the baseline.	Baseline and end of study (up to 2 years)
Number of participants with adverse events both treatment-related or not related to treatment.	To report the adverse events or risks that had to be observed carefully and registered in order to care for the safety and to accomplish regulations of any treatment or medical intervention. For this procedure, the usual risks are some adverse events as moderate to severe pain, bleeding of more than a drop, and ecchymosis bigger than 5 millimeters. Deaths and other serious events related or not with the therapeutic procedure had to be reported.	2 years

Sponsor
Escuela Neijing

Collaborators
No information provided

Investigators
- Principal Investigator: Luz H Gutierrez, MD, MPH, Escuela Neijing Colombia
- Study Director: Jose L Padilla, MD, Hispano American Acupuncture Association-Beijing 84, Madrid, Spain
- Study Chair: José R Gutiérrez, MD, Opht, Sociedad Colombiana de Oftalmología
- Study Chair: Libia V Ferrer, Tech TCM, Escuela Neijing Colombia
- Study Chair: Sergio L Pineda, Escuela Neijing Colombia

General Publications
No publications available

Results

Outcome Measures

1. Change on Visual Acuity (VA) of the Treated Eyes From Baseline to the End of
    the Study

Type: Primary|Time Frame: Baseline, 2 months and every 2 months until month 24

Description	The primary objective is to assess if acupuncture treatment is linked to a change in visual acuity (VA). VA was obtained by an ophthalmologic assessment at baseline and every two months until month 24. VA measurements were taken with the patient in a sitting position using a Snellen chart at a testing distance of 6 meters. The scale in Snellen is given in fractional numbers corresponding 20/20 to a normal vision at 20 ft or 6 meters. According to the World Health Organization, the normal vision is to 20/25, severe impairment corresponds to VA worse than 20/200 or legal blindness. Each fraction corresponds to a determined line of the chart in which all letters are correctly identified and the variation or gain is appreciated by the lines gained or lost by each eye. Improvement means a fraction better than initial, stable is no change in VA, and lost is the VA worst than those of baseline.
Time Frame	Baseline, 2 months and every 2 months until month 24.
Analysis Population Description	The primary analysis includes only patients who completed the 24-month exam. The improvement in this outcome is measured on eyes which had a vision gain in lines of the Snellen chart.

Arm/Group Title	Change in VA From Baseline to the End of Study
Arm/Group Description	There were 13 patients with neovascular AMD in one or in both eyes. The total of eyes in this condition was 22 and the other 13 participants had the dry form of AMD in one or both of their eyes, for a total of 23 eyes. This is not the sum of participants in each form of the disease because some of them had mixed conditions. Other 4 patients, 8 eyes, had macular dystrophy and 2 participants (3 eyes) had myopic degeneration. As the objective was not the comparison between them, it was prespecified to analyze them together Show more
Overall number of participants analyzed	29
Overall number of units analyzed Type of units analyzed: Eyes	56
Eyes which improved VA[a]	3664.3%

Arm/Group Title	Change in VA From Baseline to the End of Study
Eyes with stable VA[a]	1628.6%
Eyes which lost VA[a]	47.1%

[a]Unit of measure: eyes

2. **Eyes with Change From Baseline to the End of the Study in Distance Vision According to Categories CIE 10 Based on Lines Seen on the Snellen Chart.**

Type: Primary|Time Frame: 24 months from baseline

Description	Change in visual acuity was measured by the number of lines seen on the Snellen Chart from baseline to the end of the trial. The measure was obtained by an ophthalmologic assessment on both eyes at the beginning of the study and every two months until month 24 using the best correction. VA measurements (lines in which all letters are correctly identified) were performed with the patient in a sitting position using a Snellen chart at a testing distance of 6 meters and the variation is appreciated by the lines gained or lost by each eye. The measure in Snellen is given in fractional numbers. Each fraction corresponds to a determined line of the chart corresponding VA 20/20 or 6/6 to a normal vision at 20 ft or 6 meters. The range of normal vision according to the WHO is to 20/25 ft or 6/10m, Mild means VA worse than 6/12, Moderate means VA worse than 6/18, Severe means VA worse than 6/60 that is "legal blindness". Blindness is considered VA worse than 3/60.
Time Frame	24 months from baseline.
Analysis Population Description	All participants received the same treatment in a treat and extend regimen with an ophthalmological review every 2 months for 2 years. Data of VA from baseline to the end of the study were compared to assess improvement or worsening. Improved means eyes with a better score of lines, stable means equal VA, and worse is a loss of lines seen.

Arm/Group Title	VA Measured at Snellen Chart at the Beginning of the Study	VA Measured at Snellen Chart at the End of the Study
Arm/Group Description	In all participants, VA was measured at baseline. The category of visual impairment according to WHO, ICD-10	

Description	In all participants, VA was measured at baseline. The category of visual impairment according to WHO, ICD-10 is presented below. Show less	VA was measured by an ophthalmologist every 2 months. The numbers below are the final VA at 24 months from the beginning. Show less
Overall number of participants analyzed	29	29

Overall number of units analyzed Type of units analyzed: Eyes	56	56
Normal[a]	2035.7%	2951.8%
Mild[a]	35.4%	47.1%
Moderate[a]	916.1%	814.3%
Severe[a]	1933.9%	1017.9%
Blindness[a]	58.9%	58.9%

[a]Unit of measure: eyes

3. Change From Baseline in the Number of Letters Seen on the Early-Treatment Diabetic Retinopathy Study (ETDRS) Eye Chart

Type: Primary|Time Frame: Baseline and at end of study (up to 2 years)

Description	The ETDRS scale of letters is commonly used to report outcomes in AMD; for this reason, this score was chosen to compare outcomes with similar studies. Accepted tables for conversion from Snellen to ETDRS were used. Eighty-five letters are equivalent to 20/20 and 0 letters correspond to 20/200. It can be meaningful to analyze the results in this trial in the context of similar trials using anti-VEGF, or reporting a visual loss in those cases that are not treatable.
Time Frame	Baseline and at end of study (up to 2 years)
Analysis Population Description	In AMD patients, some had a form in one eye and other in the fellow. "Improved" means the eyes which improved based on the number of letters gained in the ETDRS chart over the baseline and maintained for the end of the study. "Stable" if the number of letters is almost the same and "lost" if it was reduced.

Arm/Group Title	All Eyes Which Received Acupuncture for 24 Months
Arm/Group Description	The ETDRS scale of letters is commonly used to report outcomes in AMD; for this reason, this score was chosen to compare outcomes with similar studies. Accepted tables for conversion from Snellen to ETDRS were used. There were 22 eyes diagnosed with NV AMD, 23 eyes with no NV AMD, 8 eyes with macular dystrophy, and 3 eyes with Myopic degeneration. Two eyes of all participants were excluded due to their status, one blind and one with retinal detachment. Although the observation collected the data for each macular disease form, the objective of the trial was not to compare between types of the disease and the results are grouped for the total of eyes. Show less
Overall number of participants analyzed	29
Overall number of units analyzed Type of units analyzed: eyes	56

Arm/Group Title	All Eyes Which Received Acupuncture for 24 Months
Letters seen at baseline[a]	41.5178(33.7127)
Letters seen at the end of study[a]	53.5714(30.2450)
Change from baseline[a]	14.3571(18.8684)

Statistical Analysis 1: All Eyes Which Received Acupuncture for 24 Months I Other I t-test, 1 sided
[a]Mean (Standard Deviation) I Unit of Measure: Letters on ETDRS scale

4. Number of Eyes That Improved VA From Baseline to End of the Study in Participants with Different Forms of Macular Disease Treated with Acupuncture.

Type: PrimaryITime Frame: 2 years

Description	"Improved" was defined as cases that gained in visual acuity (Note: no minimum of letters was defined). "Stable" was defined as visual acuity that did not change in the sense of not losing or gaining in the final identification of the optotypes. "Lost" was defined as patients who had a worse vision at the end than at the beginning (e.g., lost visual acuity because the disease continued its course and the treatment was not effective.)
Time Frame	2 years
Analysis Population Description	Patients with AMD can have both eyes with neovascular AMD or NV-AMD in one of the eyes and no NA-AMD in the fellow.

Arm/Group Title	Acupuncture Group Eyes With NV AMD
Arm/Group Description	Patients with neovascular membrane treated with acupuncture and massage who improved vision (AV). Therapy of Traditional Chinese Medicine (acupuncture and massage) for 24 months Acupuncture has been used for retinal diseases in hospitals of China and in other parts of the world. Some patients in this study had one or both eyes with AMD classified as Neovascular AMD by OCT and retinologist examination. In this group, 22 eyes of 13 patients were analyzed. Treatment consists of putting needles on specific points of skin one day each week initially, then with longer spaces of time according to improvement. A total of 11 Chinese needles of stainless steel, 25 x 40, were used by manual insertion and left for 12–15 min. Periocular massage is taught and is practiced daily by the patient himself or herself. Show less
Overall number of participants analyzed	13

Arm/Group Title	Acupuncture Group Eyes With NV AMD
Overall number of units analyzed Type of units analyzed: eyes	22
Measure Type: Number I Unit of Measure: eyes	13

5. Percentage of Participants Who Experienced Changes in Vision (Less Opacity, Less Distortion of Lines, Reduction of the Central Shadow)

Type: Secondary|Time Frame: Baseline and end of study (up to 2 years)

Description	At study entry, major complaints of patients were collected by survey. Participants also completed a survey at the middle and at the end of the trial. These data are the percentage of participants who reported changes to the main visual complaints that they considered significant in their lives compared with the baseline.
Time Frame	Baseline and end of study (up to 2 years)
Analysis Population Description	All the participants who had a follow-up for 24 months filled a survey about their complains and limitation in daily life at the beginning, in the middle time, and at the end of the study. The measure is the number of patients who reported improvement.

Arm/Group Title	Acupuncture Group
Arm/Group Description	Acupuncture and massage therapy of traditional Chinese medicine (acupuncture and massage) for 24 months Acupuncture and massage: Treatment consists of putting needles on specific points of skin one day each week initially, then with longer spaces of time according to improvement. A total of 11 Chinese needles of stainless steel, 25 × 40, were used by manual insertion and left for 12–15 min. Periocular massage is taught and is practiced daily by the patient himself or herself. Show less
Overall number of participants analyzed	29
Measure Type: Number I Unit of Measure: percentage of participants improved	61.45

6. Number of Participants with Adverse Events Both Treatment-related or Not
   Related to Treatment.

Type: Secondary|Time Frame: 2 years

Description	To report this measure, the adverse events or risks had to be observed carefully and registered in order to care for the safety and to accomplish regulations of any treatment or medical intervention. For this procedure, the usual risks are some adverse events as moderate to severe pain, bleeding of more than a drop, and ecchymosis bigger than 5 millimeters. Deaths and other serious events related or not with the therapeutic procedure had to be reported.
Time Frame	2 years
Analysis Population Description	Participants who suffered some adverse events as moderate to severe pain, bleeding of more than a drop, and ecchymosis bigger than 5 millimeters. Deaths and other events related or not with the therapeutic procedure.

Arm/Group Title	Adverse Events
Arm/Group Description	By law, and by the protocol of study, the adverse events were monitored. In acupuncture, the risks are not frequent and mainly they can consist of pain in the site of insertion of the needle, minimal bleeding, or ecchymosis. When the observed adverse events exceed the expectations, should have been reported, i.e., moderate to severe pain, bleeding that is more than a drop, or ecchymosis bigger than 5 millimeters in diameter. Similarly, was monitored any trouble related or not with the treatment as serious adverse events and mortality.
Overall number of participants analyzed	29
Measure Type: Number | Unit of Measure: participants	0

Adverse Events

Time Frame

Adverse events were carefully observed by 2 years

Adverse Event Reporting Description

As adverse event in acupuncture, bleeding, hematomas, and injury to vital organs
   are considered.

Arm/Group Title	All Study Participants
Arm/Group Description	Intervention: Acupuncture (Traditional Chinese Medicine) and Massage: A total of 11 Chinese needles, 25 × 40, were used by manual insertion plus periocular massage.

All-Cause Mortality

Arm/Group Title	All Study Participants
	Affected/at Risk (%)
Total	0/33 (0.00%)

Arm/Group Title	All Study Participants
Serious Adverse Events	
Arm/Group Title	All Study Participants
	Affected/at Risk (%)
Total	0/33 (0.00%)
Other (Not Including Serious) Adverse Events	
0% Frequency Threshold for Reporting Other Adverse Events	
Arm/Group Title	All Study Participants
	Affected/at Risk (%)
Total	0/33 (0.00%)

Europe

Completed

Therapeutic Potential of Omega-3 Fatty Acids Supplementation in Dry Macular Degeneration and Stargardt Disease (MADEOS)

ClinicalTrials.gov ID NCT03297515

Sponsor Ophthalmos Research and Education Institute
Information provided by Ophthalmos Research and Education Institute (Responsible Party)
Last Update Posted 2021-02-23

Study Overview

Brief Summary

Prospective, randomized, double-blind study to assess the Therapeutic Potential of Omega-3 Fatty Acids Supplementation in Dry Macular Degeneration and Stargardt Disease (Macular Degeneration Omega-3 Study—MADEOS.

Detailed Description

Age-related macular degeneration (AMD) is the leading cause of blindness in developed countries. By the year 2040, the number of people suffering from AMD is estimated to increase by 50%. Stargardt disease is the most prevalent form of macular dystrophy in children, with an estimated prevalence of 1 in 10000.

There is no effective treatment available that stops progression or improves vision in patients with dry AMD or Stargardt disease.

Considering the success in animal studies and observational human studies with omega-3 fatty acids supplementation when the blood ratio AA (arachidonic acid)/EPA (eicosapentaenoic acid) is <2, the sponsor hypothesizes that, when the blood ratio of AA/EPA is maintained below 2, the visual acuity in the group with active supplements will improve, in comparison to the control group, in patients with moderate and severe dry AMD and moderate and severe Stargardt.

Official Title
Prospective, Randomized, Double-blind Study to Assess the Therapeutic Potential
of Omega-3 Fatty Acids Supplementation in Dry Macular Degeneration and
Stargardt Disease (Macular Degeneration Omega-3 Study—MADEOS

Conditions
Dry AMD
Stargardt Disease 1

Intervention/Treatment
- Dietary Supplement: Madeos
- Dietary Supplement: Placebo

Other Study ID Numbers
- TG2017

Study Start (Actual)
2019-05-15

Primary Completion (Actual)
2020-09-22

Study Completion (Actual)
2020-09-22

Enrollment (Actual)
32

Study Type
Interventional

Phase
Not Applicable

France

Paris, France
Centre National d'Ophtalmologie des Quinze-Vingts

Germany

Gießen, Germany
Department of Ophthalmology, Justus-Liebig-University-Giessen

Italy

Chieti, Italy
Università degli Studi G. d'Annunzio Chieti-Pescara

Milan, Italy
ASST Santi Paolo e Carlo

Milan, Italy
Department of Ophthalmology, University Vita Salute

Eligibility Criteria
Description

Inclusion Criteria
- Men and women aged from 18 to 85 years old.
- Group 1: For moderate dry macular degeneration, the BCVA must be between 50 and 70 (ETDRS) at Screening Visit V1. There must be a large drusen >125 μm within 1mm from the center of the fovea. Geographic atrophy can be present, but must be >300 μm away from center of fovea;
- Group 2: For severe dry macular degeneration, the BCVA must be between 41 and 49 (ETDRS) at Screening Visit V1. Geographic atrophy can involve the fovea, but must be <2500 μm in diameter or any size GA, but >200 μm from centre of fovea anywhere;
- Group 3: For moderate Stargardt disease, the BCVA must be between 50 and 70 (ETDRS) at Screening Visit V1. The geographic area must be <2.0 mm in diameter anywhere;
- Group 4: For severe Stargardt disease, the BCVA must be between 41 and 49 (ETDRS) at Screening Visit V1. The geographic area must be <2.5 mm in diameter anywhere;
- Willingness to take the randomized trial investigational product for 6 months;
- Willingness to consent and undergo the examinations/blood testing at the visits;
- Be able to swallow large soft gel capsules;
- Take other supplements as usual; The EPA and DHA intake must be less than 1200 mg/day.

Exclusion Criteria
- Any ocular disease in either eye including: Diabetic retinopathy, Central serous retinopathy, Epiretinal membrane, Optic atrophy, Macular hole or pseudohole, Retinal vein occlusion, Amblyopia;
- Previous wet AMD in the study eye;
- Any previous ocular surgery, which may influence progression of dry macular degeneration, e.g., trabeculectomy, previous refractive surgery, pterygium surgery. Cataract surgery more than 6 months is not an exclusion criterion unless a complication has occurred during surgery;
- Any topical medication administered for other diseases such as glaucoma. Artificial tears up to 3/day will be allowed;
- Any ocular condition such as allergic conjunctivitis, moderate to severe dry eyes, scleritis, uveitis, keratitis, ocular Herpes Simplex keratitis, ectropion, entropion, ocular surface scaring;
- Any systemic conditions such as gastrointestinal disease, e.g., irritable bowel syndrome, Crohn's disease, cancer, etc.;
- Any drugs which could affect the eye administered up to 6 months before screening, e.g.: Steroids, Ethambutol, Tamoxifen, Chloroquine, Hydroxychloroquine;
- Any condition that would not allow follow-up, e.g., alcoholism or drug abuse;
- Allergy to any ingredients of the active or placebo pills.

- Pregnant or lactating;
- Current use of EPA/DHA supplements in excess of 1200 mg/day;
- History of liver disease;
- Anticoagulation therapy such as warfarin/heparin/aspirin/dabigatran/clopido-grel, etc.;
- Bleeding tendencies, e.g., coagulopathies;
- History of atrial fibrillation;
- Inability to give informed consent (impaired mental capacity, e.g., psychiatric deficit);
- Smokers or patients who have not been completely smoke free over the past 5 years.

Ages Eligible for Study
18–85 Years (Adult, Older Adult)

Sexes Eligible for Study
All

Accepts Healthy Volunteers
No

Design Details
Primary Purpose: Treatment
Allocation: Randomized
Interventional Model: Parallel Assignment
Masking: Triple (Participant Care Provider Investigator)

Arms and interventions

Participant group/arm	Intervention/treatment
Experimental: Omega 3 fatty acids Omega 3 fatty acids	Dietary Supplement: Madeos • Arm 1: Omega 3
Placebo Comparator: Placebo Placebo (sunflower oil)	Dietary Supplement: Placebo • Arm 2: Placebo

Primary outcome measures

Outcome measure	Measure description	Time frame
Mean change of letters (BCVA) from screening to 24 weeks	Mean change of letters (BCVA) from screening to 24 weeks	24 weeks

Sponsor
Ophthalmos Research and Education Institute

Collaborators
No information provided

Investigators
No information provided

General Publications
No publications available

Europe

Completed

Pupil Dynamics and Color Vision for the Detection of Eye Diseases (PupDyn)

ClinicalTrials.gov ID NCT04909398

Sponsor Centre Hospitalier National d'Ophtalmologie des Quinze-Vingts
Information provided by Centre Hospitalier National d'Ophtalmologie des Quinze-Vingts (Responsible Party)
Last Update Posted 2021-06-01

Study Overview

Brief Summary
The development of new oculometry techniques allows fine and dynamic measurements of pupillary diameter and use in routine clinical practice.

The preliminary results obtained with innovative devices on healthy subjects make it possible to envisage a clinical study on a population of patients suffering from retinal pathologies.

This is a "proof of concept" study, which, if the expected results are confirmed, will make it possible to consider a study on a larger population, as well as the industrial development of a commercial device.

Detailed Description
This is a single-head study that will take place at the National Ophthalmology Hospital Center (CHNO) and the Vision Institute (Streetlab) and the total duration of the study is 24 months.

It is planned to include 60 participants divided into different groups:

- 15 healthy subjects, called controls.
- 15 patients with retinitis pigmentosa.
- 15 patients with Leber's hereditary optic neuropathy.
- 15 patients with Stargardt's disease.

Patients will be preselected on files at the CHNO clinical investigation center based on the visual assessment carried out on the day of their arrival; the doctor may suggest that they participate in the study if the inclusion criteria are respected.

Official Title

New Methods of Dynamic Pupillometrics in Subjects with Visual and Color Vision Pathologies for the Detection, Functional Diagnosis, and Follow-up of These Pathologies

Conditions

Retinitis Pigmentosa
Leber's Hereditary Optic Neuropathy
Stargardt Disease

Intervention/Treatment

- Behavioral: Dynamic pupillometry sessions

Other Study ID Numbers

- P17-05

Study Start (Actual)

2018-03-22

Primary Completion (Actual)

2018-03-22

Study Completion (Actual)

2019-05-22

Enrollment (Actual)

60

Study Type

Interventional

Phase

Not Applicable

France

Paris, France, 75012
Centre Hospitalier National D'Ophtalùmologie des Quinze-Vingts

Eligibility Criteria
Description

Inclusion Criteria

Patients with an understanding of the French language to ensure a perfect understanding of the instructions during evaluations and documents relating to their involvement in the study.

Visually impaired volunteers:
Patients must have one of three conditions: Retinitis Pigmentosa, Stargardt disease, Leber optic neuropathy.
Healthy volunteers:

- Visual acuity of both corrected eyes (glasses) should be higher or equal 8/10th and a normal visual field.
- Patients should not wear contact lenses (which may interfere with the recording of the pupil and eye movements)

Exclusion Criteria

- Pregnant or lactating women will not be able to participate in this research.
- Participants should not be unable to personally consent.
- Subjects should not participate in another clinical trial that may interfere with this research.
- Inability to personally consent.
- Subjects should not present with degenerative diseases or any other disease that could interfere with the evaluations planned during this study.
- The subject follows a drug treatment which can cause visual disturbances, changes in pupillary kinetics, or cognitive disturbances.

Secondary exclusion criteria (at the end of the inclusion visit):

- Visually impaired subjects and controls for which calibration is not feasible.
- Patients and control subjects having difficulty maintaining visual fixation.
- Patients and subjects wearing corrective lenses, making it impossible to record oculomotor activity with an infrared camera oculometer.

Ages Eligible for Study
18–60 Years (Adult)

Sexes Eligible for Study
All

Accepts Healthy Volunteers
Yes

Design Details
Primary Purpose: Other
Allocation: N/A
Interventional Model: Single Group Assignment
Masking: None (Open Label)

Arms and interventions

Participant group/arm	Intervention/treatment

Experimental: Dynamic pupillometry sessions
It is planned to include 60 participants divided into different groups:
• 15 healthy subjects, called controls.
• 15 patients with retinitis pigmentosa.
• 15 patients with Leber's hereditary optic neuropathy.
• 15 patients with Stargardt's disease.
	Behavioral: Dynamic pupillometry sessions
	• The evaluation protocol will include the following steps:
	  – Installation of the subject, adaptation of the chin rest for the best comfort of the participant
	  – Calibration of the oculometer consisting of ocular fixation of 9 fixation points distributed on the stimulation screen
	  – Final validation of the eligibility of the subject in the study according to the success or not of the calibration.

Primary outcome measures

Outcome measure	Measure description	Time frame
Dynamic pupillometry sessions' pupillary reflex measurement	Measurement of the right eye/left eye and binocular monocular pupillary reflex: pupillary response measured for 5 s with 3 levels of screen luminance; each stimulation will be separated from the next by a delay of 5 s	Week 1
RAPD measurement	Alternate stimulation of the right and left eye: 10 repetitions, each corresponding to the stimulation of one eye for one second.	Week 1
Endogenous pupillary oscillation measurement	Pupil oscillation frequency, for each eye and in binocular: during this test, the participants observe the stimulation screen (central fixation point) for 45 s during which the luminance of the screen is calculated to be proportional to the size of the pupil in real time.	Week 1
Measurement of pupillary activity by frequency marking	This test consists of the simultaneous presentation of 5 areas of the screen, each of which is luminance modulated at a specific frequency.	Week 1
Pupillary measurement of color vision	In this test, 2 background colors alternate at low frequency over time. The physical luminance of one color is fixed, while the other is adaptively changed during a test to reduce pupillary response.	Week 1

Sponsor

Centre Hospitalier National d'Ophtalmologie des Quinze-Vingts

Collaborators

• Streetlab

Investigators

• Principal Investigator: Saddek MOHAND-SAID, Centre Hospitalier National d'Ophtalmologie des Quinze-Vingts

General Publications

No publications available

United Kingdom

Completed

A Follow-Up Study to Determine the Safety and Tolerability of Subretinal Transplantation of Human Embryonic Stem Cell-Derived Retinal Pigmented Epithelial (hESC-RPE) Cells in Patients with Stargardt's Macular Dystrophy (SMD)

ClinicalTrials.gov ID NCT02941991

Sponsor Astellas Institute for Regenerative Medicine
Information provided by Astellas Pharma Inc (Astellas Institute for Regenerative Medicine) (Responsible Party)
Last Update Posted 2020-12-10

Study Overview

Brief Summary
The purpose of this study is to evaluate the long-term safety and tolerability of hESC-RPE cellular therapy in patients with advanced SMD from 1 to 5 years following the surgical procedure to implant the hESC-RPE cells.

Detailed Description
This study is a long-term, follow-up of a Phase I/II, open-label, non-randomized, 4-cohort, dose escalation, multicenter clinical trial (referred to as the core trial or core protocol) in which a maximum of 12 SMD patients were transplanted with sequential doses of hESC-RPE cells, starting at a dose of 50,000 hESC-RPE cells transplanted and increasing to a maximum dose of 200,000 hESC-RPE cells transplanted. All patients who participate in the core protocol are eligible for participation in the follow-up protocol. The first visit of this extension protocol will correspond to the last visit of the core protocol and will take place at 12 months post-cell implantation. Informed consent for this follow-up protocol will be obtained at the first visit which will occur at the 12-month visit of the core protocol. Patients will be evaluated at 18, 24, 36, 48, and 60 months posttransplant (or more frequently as clinically indicated). Follow-up will include obtaining information about ophthalmological findings and events of special interest as defined in the primary outcome. At the last visit of this follow-up study, whether at 60 months posttransplant or at early discontinuation, patients will be invited to participate in a lifelong annual health survey, under a separate protocol, to further monitor long-term safety.

Official Title
Follow-up to 5 Years of a Phase I/II, Open-Label, Multicenter, Prospective Study to Determine the Safety and Tolerability of Subretinal Transplantation of Human Embryonic Stem Cell-Derived Retinal Pigmented Epithelial (hESC-RPE) Cells in Patients With Stargardt's Macular Dystrophy (SMD)

Conditions
Stargardt's Macular Dystrophy

Intervention/Treatment
* Biological: hESC-RPE

Other Study ID Numbers
* 7316-CL-0006
* 2012-002827-14 (EudraCT Number)
* ACT-hESC-RPE-SMD-01FU EU (Other Identifier) (OTHER: Sponsor)

Study Start (Actual)
2013-01-16

Primary Completion (Actual)
2019-10-02

Study Completion (Actual)
2019-10-02

Enrollment (Actual)
12

Study Type
Observational

United Kingdom

London, United Kingdom, EC1V2PD
Moorfields Eye Hospital NHS Foundation Trust

Newcastle upon Tyne, United Kingdom, NE7 7DN
Newcastle on Tyne NHS Foundation Trust

Eligibility Criteria
Description

Inclusion Criteria
* Must have been treated with hESC-RPE cell transplant in the core protocol.
* Able to understand and willing to sign the informed consent to participate in the follow-up study.

Exclusion Criteria
* There are no exclusion criteria

Study Population
The study population is by invitation only from previous participants in the core protocol.

Ages Eligible for Study
18 Years and older (Adult, Older Adult)

Sexes Eligible for Study
All

Accepts Healthy Volunteers
No
Sampling Method
Non-Probability Sample

Design Details
Observational Model: Cohort
Time Perspective: Prospective

Cohorts and interventions

Group/cohort	Intervention/treatment
Uniocular subretinal injection of hESC-RPE cells Cohort 1. 50,000 cells transplanted; Cohort 2. 100,000 cells transplanted; Cohort 3. 150,000 cells transplanted; Cohort 4. 200,000 cells transplanted	Biological: hESC-RPE • subretinal injection • Other Names: – ASP7316

Primary outcome measures

Outcome measure	Measure description	Time frame
Safety assessed by Adverse Events (AEs) of special interest in regard to the investigational product	This will include obtaining information about Serious Adverse Events (SAEs) that are neurologic, infectious, hematologic, or fatal; any Adverse Event (AE) that causes the subject to withdraw from the study, any new diagnosis of an ocular or immune-mediated disorder, cancer (irrespective of prior history), ectopic or proliferative cell growth (Retinal pigment epithelium (RPE) or non-RPE) with adverse clinical consequence, unexpected, clinically significant AE possibly related to the cell transplant procedure or the investigational product (hESC-RPE cells), pregnancy in a female subject or the partner of a male subject, and pregnancy outcome.	4 years

Secondary outcome measures

Outcome measure	Measure description	Time frame
Incidence of graft failure or rejection	Evidence of graft failure or rejection may consist of: Presence of retinal edema, cystoid macular edema, retinal white dots, retinal hemorrhage, serous retinal detachment, subretinal exudates, subretinal fibrosis, ocular vascular and/ or optic disc leakage, and elevated intraocular pressure or hypotony. Evidence of unanticipated and persistent or increasing noninfectious ocular inflammation (e.g., vasculitis, retinitis, choroiditis, vitritis, pars planitis, anterior segment inflammation/uveitis).	4 years

Outcome measure	Measure description	Time frame
Number of patients with changes in ocular examinations or images	The number of patients with clinically significant absolute values or changes from baseline in Intraocular pressure (IOP) and Best-Corrected Visual Acuity (BCVA) will be summarized.	4 years

Sponsor
Astellas Institute for Regenerative Medicine

Collaborators
No information provided

Investigators
- Study Director: Medical Director, Astellas Institute for Regenerative Medicine

General Publications
No publications available

United Kingdom

Completed

Safety and Tolerability of Subretinal Transplantation of Human Embryonic Stem Cell-Derived Retinal Pigmented Epithelial (hESC-RPE) Cells in Patients with Stargardt's Macular Dystrophy (SMD)

ClinicalTrials.gov ID NCT01469832

Sponsor Astellas Institute for Regenerative Medicine
Information provided by Astellas Pharma Inc (Astellas Institute for Regenerative Medicine) (Responsible Party)
Last Update Posted 2021-07-07

Study Overview

Brief Summary
The purpose of this study is:
To evaluate the safety and tolerability of RPE cellular therapy in patients with SMD.
To evaluate potential efficacy endpoints to be used in future studies of RPE cellular therapy.

Detailed Description
This study is a Phase I/II, open-label, non-randomized, sequential, multicenter clinical trial.

There will be 5 cohorts; the 4 low vision cohorts will contain 3 patients, the better vision cohort will contain 4 patients. The enrolled cohorts will be as follows:

Three SMD patients- 50,000 MA09-hRPE cells transplanted
Three SMD patients- 100,000 MA09-hRPE cells transplanted
Four Better Vision SMD patients- 100,000 MA09-hRPE cells transplanted
Three SMD patients- 150,000 MA09-hRPE cells transplanted
Three SMD patients- 200,000 MA09-hRPE cells transplanted

Patients will be enrolled sequentially, and within each cohort of 3 patients, each patient's clinical course over the first 6 weeks following cell transplantation will be reviewed by an independent DSMB before enrollment is opened for the next 2 patients. A full safety assessment of all 3 patients in each cohort will be made by the DSMB when the 3rd patient in each cohort completes 4 weeks of follow-up, and before the first patient in the next cohort receives a cell transplant. The exception is the better vision group where all patients may be enrolled once DSMB approval has been received.

Each cohort will be enrolled sequentially in turn, with the exception of the better vision cohort which may be enrolled in parallel with the other cohorts.

The day of the cell implantation will be Day 0, and patients will remain in the study until the last visit at 12 months.

Official Title

A Phase I/II, Open-Label, Multicenter, Prospective Study to Determine the Safety and Tolerability of Subretinal Transplantation of Human Embryonic Stem Cell-Derived Retinal Pigmented Epithelial (hESC-RPE) Cells in Patients With Stargardt's Macular Dystrophy (SMD)

Conditions

Stargardt's Macular Dystrophy

Intervention/Treatment

- Biological: MA09-hRPE

Other Study ID Numbers

- 7316-CL-0003
- 2011-000054-34 (EudraCT Number)
- ACT hESC-RPE SMD 01 EU (Other Identifier) (OTHER: Sponsor)

Study Start (Actual)

2011-12-13

Primary Completion (Actual)

2015-09-30

Study Completion (Actual)

2015-09-30

Enrollment (Actual)

12

Study Type
Interventional

Phase
Phase 1 and Phase 2

United Kingdom

Edinburgh, United Kingdom, EH1 3EG
Lothian Health Board Headquarters at Waverley Gate

London, United Kingdom, EC1V2PD
Moorfields Eye Hospital NHS Foundation Trust

Newcastle upon Tyne, United Kingdom, NE7 7DN
Newcastle on Tyne NHS Foundation Trust

Eligibility Criteria
Description

Inclusion Criteria
- Adult male or female over 18 years of age. Clinical diagnosis of SMD: If known, the patient's genotype will be recorded in the medical history; if unknown, patient will allow for the submission of a sample for genotyping.

Independently verified clinical findings consistent with SMD: The visual acuity of the eye to receive the transplant will be no better than 20/400. The visual acuity of the eye in the better vision cohort to receive the transplant will be no better than 20/100.

The visual acuity of the eye that is not to receive the transplant will be no better than 20/400 for the worse vision patients and no worse than 20/100 for the better vision patients.

Electrophysiological findings consistent with SMD: Medically suitable to undergo vitrectomy and subretinal injection. Medically suitable for general anesthesia or waking sedation, if needed.

Medically suitable for transplantation of an embryonic stem cell line:

- Normal serum chemistry (sequential multichannel analyzer 20 [SMA-20]) and hematology (complete blood count [CBC], prothrombin time [PT], and activated partial thromboplastin time [aPTT]) screening tests.
- Negative urine screen for drugs of abuse.
- Negative human immunodeficiency virus (HIV), hepatitis B (HBV), and hepatitis C (HCV) serologies.
- No history of malignancy, with the exception of successfully treated basal cell or squamous cell carcinoma of the skin.
- Negative cancer screening within previous 6 months:

Complete history and physical examination; dermatological screening exam for malignant lesions; negative fecal occult blood test negative chest roentgenogram (CXR); normal CBC & manual differential; negative urinalysis (U/A); normal thyroid exam and thyroid panel; if male, normal testicular examination; if over age 40, digital rectal examination (DRE) and prostate-specific antigen (PSA); if female, normal pelvic examination with Papanicolaou smear; and if female, normal clinical breast exam; and if 50 years of age or older, negative mammogram.

If female and of childbearing potential, willing to use an effective form of birth control during the study.

If male, willing to use barrier and spermicide contraception during the study. Willing to defer all future blood, blood component, or tissue donation. Able to understand and willing to sign the informed consent.

Exclusion Criteria
- History of malignancy, with the exception of successfully treated basal cell or squamous cell carcinoma of the skin.

History of myocardial infarction in previous 12 months. History of diabetes mellitus. Any immunodeficiency. Any current immunosuppressive therapy other than intermittent or low-dose corticosteroids.

Serologic evidence of infection with Hepatitis B, Hepatitis C, or HIV. Current participation in any other clinical trial. Participation within previous 6 months in any clinical trial of a drug by ocular or systemic administration.

Any other sight-threatening ocular disease. Any chronic ocular medications. Any history of retinal vascular disease (compromised blood-retinal barrier). Glaucoma. Uveitis or other intraocular inflammatory disease. Significant lens opacities or other media opacity. Ocular lens removal within previous 3 months.

Ages Eligible for Study
18 Years and older (Adult, Older Adult)

Sexes Eligible for Study
All

Accepts Healthy Volunteers
No

Design Details
Primary Purpose: Treatment
Allocation: N/A
Interventional Model: Single Group Assignment
Masking: None (Open Label)

Arms and interventions

Participant group/arm	Intervention/treatment
Experimental: Subretinal injection of MA09-hRPE • Cohort 1 50,000 cells • Cohort 2 100,000 cells • Cohort 2a Better Vision 100,000 cells • Cohort 3 150,000 cells • Cohort 4 200,000 cells	Biological: MA09-hRPE – Cohort 1 50,000 cells – Cohort 2 100,000 cells – Cohort 2a Better Vision 100,000 cells – Cohort 3 150,000 cells – Cohort 4 200,000 cells

Primary outcome measures

Outcome measure	Measure description	Time frame
Safety and tolerance of transplantation	The safety and tolerance of transplantation of hESC-derived MA09-hRPE will be considered safe and tolerated in the absence of: Any grade 2 NCI grading system or greater adverse event related to the cell product. Any evidence that the cells are contaminated with an infectious agent or have tumorigenic potential, Adverse Event and Serious Adverse Event assessment, Serial vital signs and Clinical laboratory tests, Direct ophthalmological monitoring of RPE cells' acceptance/integrity/rejection, Monitoring of local and systemic infection or tumorigenic cell transformation	12 months

Secondary outcome measures

Outcome measure	Measure description	Time frame
Evidence of successful engraftment	• Evidence of successful engraftment. Evidence of successful engraftment will consist of: • Structural evidence (OCT imaging, fluorescein angiography, autofluorescence photography, slit-lamp examination with fundus photography) that cells have been implanted in the correct location • Electroretinographic evidence (mfERG) showing enhanced activity in the implant location	12 months

Sponsor

Astellas Institute for Regenerative Medicine

Collaborators

No information provided

Investigators

• Study Director: Medical Director, Astellas Institute for Regenerative Medicine

General Publications

• Schwartz SD, Hubschman JP, Heilwell G, Franco-Cardenas V, Pan CK, Ostrick RM, Mickunas E, Gay R, Klimanskaya I, Lanza R. Embryonic stem cell trials for macular degeneration: a preliminary report. Lancet. 2012 Feb 25;379(9817):713–20. https://doi.org/10.1016/S0140-6736(12)60028-2. Epub 2012 Jan 24.

• Schwartz SD, Regillo CD, Lam BL, Eliott D, Rosenfeld PJ, Gregori NZ, Hubschman JP, Davis JL, Heilwell G, Spirn M, Maguire J, Gay R, Bateman J, Ostrick RM, Morris D, Vincent M, Anglade E, Del Priore LV, Lanza R. Human embryonic stem cell-derived retinal pigment epithelium in patients with age-related macular degeneration and Stargardt's macular dystrophy: follow-up of two open-label phase 1/2 studies. Lancet. 2015 Feb 7;385(9967):509–16. https://doi.org/10.1016/S0140-6736(14)61376-3. Epub 2014 Oct 15.

No Location

Completed

Phase 1 Safety Study of ALK-001 in Healthy Volunteers

ClinicalTrials.gov ID NCT02230228

Sponsor Alkeus Pharmaceuticals, Inc.
Information provided by Alkeus Pharmaceuticals, Inc. (Responsible Party)
Last Update Posted 2015-03-24

Study Overview

Brief Summary
This protocol is a phase 1 clinical study to assess the safety and pharmacokinetics of ALK-001 in healthy volunteers. Please contact trials@alkeus.com for any questions.

Official Title
A Phase 1, Open-Label, Repeat Dose Study to Investigate the Safety and Pharmacokinetics of 4-week Daily Dosing of ALK-001 in Healthy Volunteers

Conditions
Stargardt Disease
Age-related Macular Degeneration
Other Retinal Dystrophies

Intervention/Treatment
• Drug: ALK-001 (No generic name)

Other Study ID Numbers
• ALK001-P1001

Study Start
2014-04

Primary Completion (Actual)
2014-09

Study Completion (Actual)
2015-02

Enrollment (Actual)
40

Study Type
Interventional

Phase
Phase 1

Eligibility Criteria
Description

Main Inclusion Criteria
- Adult between 21 and 70 years old (inclusive)
- Healthy subject, as judged by investigator
- Subject is able and willing to comply with study requirements (study medication compliance, schedule of follow-up visits)
- Subject has provided informed consent to participate
- If female, subject uses a medically accepted birth control method and agrees to use such a method for entire clinical trial period

Main Exclusion Criteria
- Subject has taken disallowed items during the past 30 days
- Female with a positive urine pregnancy test at screening
- Lactating woman
- Subject has participated in any clinical study involving an investigational drug, biologic or device, during the past 30 days
- History or current evidence of gastrointestinal malabsorption
- Subject has any other medical condition, which, in the opinion of the investigator, is likely to prevent compliance with protocol and/or interfere with successful collection of study
- Subject has, in the opinion of investigator, clinically significant laboratory result(s), positive drug or alcohol screening, or ECG, which makes subject unsuitable for participation.

Ages Eligible for Study
21–70 Years (Adult, Older Adult)

Sexes Eligible for Study
All

Accepts Healthy Volunteers
Yes

Design Details
Primary Purpose: Basic Science
Allocation: N/A
Interventional Model: Single Group Assignment
Masking: None (Open Label)

Arms and interventions

Participant group/arm	Intervention/treatment

Experimental: ALK-001 capsules	Drug: ALK-001 (No generic name)
	• Daily, oral administration of ALK-001 capsules.
	• Other Names:
	  – C20-D3-Retinyl Acetate
	  – C20 Deuterated vitamin A

Primary outcome measures

Outcome measure	Measure description	Time frame
Safety of 4-week daily dosing of ALK-001 in healthy adults.	Safety evaluations combine: adverse events (AE), laboratory testing (hematology and biochemistry panels), 12-lead electrocardiograms (ECGs), vital signs, physical examination, and visual function (visual acuity and a self-reported questionnaire).	4 weeks

Sponsor
Alkeus Pharmaceuticals, Inc.

Collaborators
No information provided

Investigators
- Study Director: Leonide Saad, PhD, Alkeus Pharmaceuticals, Inc.
- Study Chair: Ilyas Washington, PhD, Columbia University

General Publications
No publications available

Chapter 7
Terminated Studies

United States

Reason: Study stopped not for safety reasons. Due to review of clinical development plans and priorities, sponsor decided to stop development of the product.

Phase I/IIA Study of SAR422459 in Participants with Stargardt's Macular Degeneration

ClinicalTrials.gov ID NCT01367444

Sponsor Sanofi
Information provided by Sanofi (Responsible Party)
Last Update Posted 2022-04-14

Brief Summary
Primary Objective
To assess the safety and tolerability of ascending doses of SAR422459 in participants with Stargardt's Macular Degeneration (SMD).

Secondary Objective
To evaluate for possible biological activity of SAR422459.

Detailed Description
The total duration per participant was up to 52 weeks, which included 4-week screening period and 48-weeks study period.

At the end of the study, the participants were invited to enter in an open-label safety study (LTS13588-NCT01736592) for long-term follow-up visits including ophthalmological examinations and recording of adverse events (AEs) for up to 15 years.

© The Author(s), under exclusive license to Springer Nature Switzerland AG 2024

J. N. Weiss, *Clinical Trials in Stargardt Disease Treatment*,
https://doi.org/10.1007/978-3-031-58807-5_7

Official Title
A Phase I/IIA Dose Escalation Safety Study of Subretinally Injected SAR422459,
   Administered to Patients With Stargardt's Macular Degeneration

Conditions
Stargardt's Disease

Intervention/Treatment
• Drug: SAR422459

Other Study ID Numbers
• TDU13583
• SG1/001/10

Study Start (Actual)
2011-06-08

Primary Completion (Actual)
2019-08-16

Study Completion (Actual)
2019-08-16

Enrollment (Actual)
27

Study Type
Interventional

Phase
Phase 1 and Phase 2

United States
Florida Locations

Miami, Florida, United States, 33136
Investigational Site Number 840002

Iowa Locations

Iowa City, Iowa, United States, 52242
Investigational Site Number 840005

Oregon Locations

Portland, Oregon, United States, 97239-3098
Investigational Site Number 840001

Texas Locations

Houston, Texas, United States, 77030
Investigational Site Number 840004

France

Paris, France, 75012
Investigational Site Number 250001

Inclusion Criteria

- Signed and dated written informed consent obtained from the participant and/or the participant's legally acceptable representative.
- Diagnosis of SMD, with at least one pathogenic mutant ABCA4 allele on each chromosome.
- Women of childbearing potential must have a negative pregnancy test at Day -1 and agree to use an effective form of contraception for at least three months, or be surgically sterile or postmenopausal, with the last menstrual period being over two years prior to enrollment.
- Males must agree with their partner to use two forms of contraception for at least three months following SAR422459 administration.
- Participants must agree to not donate blood, organs, tissues, or cells for at least three months following SAR422459 administration.
- Participants enrolled in France must be affiliated to or benefit from a social security regimen.

Specific Inclusion Criteria Participant Group A

- Participants (18 years or older) with advanced SMD.
- Visual acuity less than or equal to (<=) 20/200 in the worst eye.
- Severe cone-rod dysfunction with no detectable or severely abnormal full-field electroretinogram responses.

Specific Inclusion Criteria Participant Group B

- Participants (18 years or older) with SMD.
- Visual Acuity <=20/200 in the worst eye.
- Abnormal full-field electroretinogram responses.

Specific Inclusion Criteria Participant Group C

- Participants (18 years or older) with SMD.
- Visual acuity <=20/100 in the worst eye.
- Abnormal full-field electroretinogram responses.

Specific Inclusion Criteria Participant Group D

- Symptomatic participants (from 6 years to 26 years old) with early or childhood-onset SMD (age at disease onset [less than] <18 years) with at least one pathogenic mutant ABCA4 allele on each chromosome confirmed by direct sequencing and co-segregation analysis within the participant's family.
- Visual acuity of greater than or equal to (>=) 20/200 in both eyes at the time of the screening visit.
- Participants were anticipated to experience rapid deterioration in visual function and/or retinal structure as determined by an annual progression rate in at least one of the following parameters occurring in at least one eye (assessments recorded up to 2 years prior to the screening visit date might be considered to document evidence of rapid deterioration):

- Loss of >=1 line of Snellen visual acuity (equivalent to 5 early treatment diabetic retinopathy study [ETDRS] letters).
- Reduction in macular mean sensitivity of >=1.2 decibels (dB) as assessed by microperimetry.
- Reduction in macular mean sensitivity of >=5 dB or reduction in hill of vision by greater than (>)14 dB-sr as assessed by static perimetry.
- Enlargement in the area of macular retinal pigment epithelial (RPE) atrophy by fundus autofluorescence at a rate of >=0.5 millimeter square (mm^2).
- Enlargement in the area of central macular retinal thinning/photoreceptor loss by ocular coherence tomography at a rate of >=0.5 mm^2.

- All eligible participants must demonstrate an ability to understand, willingness to cooperate, and ability to reliably perform required study procedures as judged and confirmed by the study investigator.

Specific Inclusion Criteria Participant Group E
- Symptomatic participants (between 6 years and 17 years old) with early or childhood-onset SMD with at least one pathogenic mutant ABCA4 allele on each chromosome confirmed by direct sequencing and co-segregation analysis within the participant's family.
- Visual acuity of >=20/100 in both eyes at the time of screening visit.
- Participants were anticipated to experience rapid deterioration in visual function and/or retinal structure as determined by an annual progression rate in at least one of the following parameters occurring in at least one eye (assessments recorded up to 2 years prior to the screening visit date were considered to document evidence of rapid deterioration):

- Loss of >=1 line of Snellen visual acuity (equivalent to 5 ETDRS letters).
- Reduction in macular mean sensitivity of >=1.2 dB as assessed by microperimetry.
- Reduction in macular mean sensitivity of >=5 dB or reduction in hill of vision by >14 dB-sr as assessed by static perimetry.
- Enlargement in the area of macular RPE atrophy by fundus autofluorescence at a rate of >=0.5 mm^2.
- Enlargement in the area of central macular retinal thinning/photoreceptor loss by ocular coherence tomography at a rate of >=0.5 mm^2.

- All eligible participants demonstrated an ability to understand, willingness to cooperate, and ability to reliably perform required study procedures as judged and confirmed by the study investigator.

Exclusion Criteria
- Preexisting eye conditions that would preclude the planned surgery or interfere with the interpretation of study outcome measures.
- Cataract surgery with intraocular lens implantation within 6 months of enrolment.
- Aphakia or prior vitrectomy in the study eye.
- Concomitant systemic diseases including those in which the disease itself, or the treatment for the disease, can alter ocular function.

- Any intraocular surgery or laser in either eye planned within 6 months of Day 0.
- Any contraindication to pupil dilation in either eye.
- Any known allergy to any component of the delivery vehicle or diagnostic agents used during the study, or medications planned for use in the perioperative period particularly topical, injected, or systemic corticosteroids.
- Any injectable intravitreal treatment to the treated eye or intravitreal device in the treated eye within 6 months prior to screening.
- Any periocular injections of corticosteroids to the treated eye within 4 months prior to screening.
- Laboratory test abnormalities or abnormalities in electrocardiogram, chest X-rays that in the opinion of the principal investigator would make the participant unsuitable for participation in the study.
- Significant intercurrent illness or infection during the 28 days prior to enrolment.
- Premenopausal or nonsurgically sterile women who were unwilling to use an effective form of contraception such as the contraceptive pill or intrauterine device.
- Alcohol or other substance abuse.
- Contraindications to use of anesthesia (local or general, as appropriate).
- Concurrent antiretroviral therapy that would inactivate the investigational agent.
- History of any investigational agent within 28 days prior to SAR422459 administration.
- Participation in a prior ocular gene transfer therapy study.
- Enrolment in any other clinical treatment study throughout the duration of the SAR422459 study.
- Current or anticipated treatment with anticoagulant therapy or the use of anticoagulation therapy within the four weeks prior to surgery.
- A past medical history of human immunodeficiency virus or hepatitis A, B, or C infection.
- Women who were pregnant or were breastfeeding.
- History or signs consistent with unilateral amblyopia (strabismic, anisometropic, or stimulus deprivation).

Ages Eligible for Study
6 Years and older (Child, Adult, Older Adult)

Sexes Eligible for Study
All

Accepts Healthy Volunteers
No

Design Details
Primary Purpose: Treatment
Allocation: Non-Randomized
Interventional Model: Single Group Assignment
Masking: None (Open Label)

Arms and interventions

Participant group/arm	Intervention/treatment
Experimental: SAR422459 (Dose 1) Starting dose of SAR422459 given through subretinal injection	Drug: SAR422459 • Pharmaceutical form: sterile solution, 100 microliters (µL) aliquots in 0.3 milliliter (mL) type I borosilicate glass 'V' vials with a butyl stopper and aluminum crimp seal. Route of administration: subretinal injection
Experimental: SAR422459 (Dose 2) Escalating dose of SAR422459 given through subretinal injection	Drug: SAR422459 • Pharmaceutical form: sterile solution, 100 microliters (µL) aliquots in 0.3 milliliter (mL) type I borosilicate glass 'V' vials with a butyl stopper and aluminum crimp seal. Route of administration: subretinal injection
Experimental: SAR422459 (Dose 3) Maximum tolerated dose (MTD) of SAR422459 given through subretinal injection	Drug: SAR422459 • Pharmaceutical form: sterile solution, 100 microliters (µL) aliquots in 0.3 milliliter (mL) type I borosilicate glass 'V' vials with a butyl stopper and aluminum crimp seal. Route of administration: subretinal injection

Primary outcome measures

Outcome measure	Measure description	Time frame
Percentage of Participants With Treatment-emergent Adverse Events (TEAEs)	An adverse event (AE) was any unfavorable and unintended physical sign, symptom, or laboratory parameter that developed or worsened in severity during the course of the study, whether or not considered related to the investigational product. The TEAEs were defined as any event that started or increased in severity after the participant received investigational medicinal product (IMP), including abnormal laboratory results, electrocardiogram, etc.	From Baseline to Week 48
Percentage of Participants With TEAEs by Severity	An AE was any unfavorable and unintended physical sign, symptom, or laboratory parameter that developed or worsened in severity during the course of the study, whether or not considered related to the investigational product. For each AE, the severity was categorized as either mild, moderate, or severe, where 'mild' was defined as discomfort noticed but did not interfere with the participant's daily routines (an annoyance), 'moderate' was defined as some impairment of function, not hazardous to health (uncomfortable or embarrassing), and 'severe' was defined as significant impairment of function, hazardous to health (incapacitating).	From Baseline to Week 48

Sponsor
Sanofi

Collaborators
No information provided

Investigators
- Principal Investigator: Paul Yang, MD, Oregon Health & Science University, Portland, Oregon
- Principal Investigator: Jose-Alain Sahel, MD. Ph.D, Hopital Nationale des Quinze-Vingt, Paris France

General Publications
No publications available

Results

Outcome Measures

1. Percentage of Participants with Treatment-Emergent Adverse Events (TEAEs)

Type: Primary|Time Frame: From Baseline to Week 48

Description	An adverse event (AE) was any unfavorable and unintended physical sign, symptom, or laboratory parameter that developed or worsened in severity during the course of the study, whether or not considered related to the investigational product. The TEAEs were defined as any event that started or increased in severity after the participant received investigational medicinal product (IMP), including abnormal laboratory results, electrocardiogram, etc.
Time Frame	From Baseline to Week 48
Analysis Population Description	Analysis was performed on all participants with SMD who were included in the study.

Arm/Group Title	Cohort 1	Cohort 2	Cohort 3	Cohort 4	Cohort 5	Cohort 6	Cohort 7
Arm/Group Description	Participants (aged >=18 years) with advanced SMD, and VA <=20/200 in the worst eye and severe cone-rod dysfunction with no detectable or severely abnormal full-field ERG responses, received SAR422459 at lowest target dose level 1.8*10^5 TU/study eye. Show less	Participants (aged >=18 years) with SMD, and VA <=20/200 in the worst eye with abnormal full-field ERG responses, received SAR422459 at lowest target dose level 1.8*10^5 TU/study eye. Show less	Participants (aged >=18 years) with SMD, and VA <=20/200 in the worst eye with abnormal full-field ERG responses, received SAR422459 at escalated target dose level 6*10^5 TU/study eye. Show less	Participants (aged >=18 years) with SMD, and VA <=20/200 in the worst eye with abnormal full-field ERG responses, received SAR422459 at target dose level 1.8*10^6 TU/study eye. Show less	Participants (aged >=18 years) with SMD, and VA <=20/100 in the worst eye with abnormal full-field ERG responses, received SAR422459 at highest target dose level 1.8*10^6 TU/study eye. Show less	Participants (aged 6 to 26 years) with symptomatic early or childhood-onset SMD, and VA >=20/200 in both eyes at the time of the screening visit and anticipated to experience rapid deterioration in visual function and/or retinal structure, received SAR422459 at highest target dose level 1.8*10^6 TU/study eye. Show less	Pediatric participants (aged 6–17 years) with symptomatic SMD, and VA >=20/100 in both eyes at the time of the screening visit and anticipated to experience rapid deterioration in visual function and/or retinal structure, received SAR422459 at highest target dose level 1.8*10^6 TU/study eye. Show less
Overall Number of Participants Analyzed	4	4	4	4	6	4	1
Measure Type: Number | Unit of Measure: Percentage of Participants	100	100	100	100	100	100	100

2. Percentage of Participants with TEAEs by Severity

Type: Primary|Time Frame: From Baseline to Week 48

Description	An AE was any unfavorable and unintended physical sign, symptom, or laboratory parameter that developed or worsened in severity during the course of the study, whether or not considered related to the investigational product. For each AE, the severity was categorized as either mild, moderate, or severe, where 'mild' was defined as discomfort noticed but did not interfere with the participant's daily routines (an annoyance), 'moderate' was defined as some impairment of function, not hazardous to health (uncomfortable or embarrassing), and 'severe' was defined as significant impairment of function, hazardous to health (incapacitating).
Time Frame	From Baseline to Week 48
Analysis Population Description	Analysis was performed on all participants with SMD who were included in the study.

Arm/Group Title	Cohort 1	Cohort 2	Cohort 3	Cohort 4	Cohort 5	Cohort 6	Cohort 7
Arm/Group Description	Participants (aged >=18 years) with advanced SMD, and VA <=20/200 in the worst eye and severe cone-rod dysfunction with no detectable or severely abnormal full-field ERG responses, received SAR422459 at lowest target dose level 1.8*10^5 TU/study eye. Show less	Participants (aged >=18 years) with SMD, and VA <=20/200 in the worst eye with abnormal full-field ERG responses, received SAR422459 at lowest target dose level 1.8*10^5 TU/study eye. Show less	Participants (aged >=18 years) with SMD, and VA <=20/200 in the worst eye with abnormal full-field ERG responses, received SAR422459 at escalated target dose level 6*10^5 TU/study eye. Show less	Participants (aged >=18 years) with SMD, and VA <=20/200 in the worst eye with abnormal full-field ERG responses, received SAR422459 at target dose level 1.8*10^6 TU/ study eye. Show less	Participants (aged >=18 years) with SMD, and VA <=20/100 in the worst eye with abnormal full-field ERG responses, received SAR422459 at highest target dose level 1.8*10^6 TU/ study eye. Show less	Participants (aged 6 to 26 years) with symptomatic early or childhood-onset SMD, and VA >=20/200 in both eyes at the time of the screening visit and anticipated to experience rapid deterioration in visual function and/or retinal structure, received SAR422459 at highest target dose level 1.8*10^6 TU/study eye. Show less	Pediatric participants (aged 6–17 years) with symptomatic SMD, and VA >=20/100 in both eyes at the time of the screening visit and anticipated to experience rapid deterioration in visual function and/or retinal structure, received SAR422459 at highest target dose level 1.8*10^6 TU/study eye. Show less
Overall Number of Participants Analyzed	4	4	4	4	6	4	1
Mild	100	100	100	100	100	100	100
Moderate[a]	0	50	25	25	33	75	100
Severe[a]	0	0	0	25	17	25	0

[a]Measure Type: Number | Unit of Measure: percentage of participants

Adverse Events

Time Frame

All AEs were collected from time of first dose of study drug up to end of study (Week 48) regardless of seriousness or relationship (causality) to IMP.

Adverse Event Reporting Description

Reported AEs were TEAEs that developed/worsened during the 'on treatment period' (from Day 0 to Week 48). Analysis was performed on all participants with SMD who were included in the study.

ARM/Group Title	Cohort 1	Cohort 2	Cohort 3	Cohort 4	Cohort 5	Cohort 6	Cohort 7
Arm/Group Description	Participants (aged >=18 years) with advanced SMD, and VA <=20/200 in the worst eye and severe cone-rod dysfunction with no detectable or severely abnormal full-field ERG responses, received SAR422459 at lowest target dose level 1.8*10^5 TU/study eye. Show less	Participants (aged >=18 years) with SMD, and VA <=20/200 in the worst eye with abnormal full-field ERG responses, received SAR422459 at lowest target dose level 1.8*10^5 TU/ study eye. Show less	Participants (aged >=18 years) with SMD, and VA <=20/200 in the worst eye with abnormal full-field ERG responses, received SAR422459 at escalated target dose level 6*10^5 TU/ study eye. Show less	Participants (aged >=18 years) with SMD, and VA <=20/200 in the worst eye with abnormal full-field ERG responses, received SAR422459 at target dose level 1.8*10^6 TU/ study eye. Show less	Participants (aged >=18 years) with SMD, and VA <=20/100 in the worst eye with abnormal full-field ERG responses, received SAR422459 at highest target dose level 1.8*10^6 TU/ study eye. Show less	Participants (aged 6–26 years) with symptomatic early or childhood-onset SMD, and VA >=20/200 in both eyes at the time of the screening visit and anticipated to experience rapid deterioration in visual function and/ or retinal structure, received SAR422459 at highest target dose level 1.8*10^6 TU/ study eye. Show less	Pediatric participants (aged 6–17 years) with symptomatic SMD, and VA >=20/100 in both eyes at the time of the screening visit and anticipated to experience rapid deterioration in visual function and/or retinal structure, received SAR422459 at highest target dose level 1.8*10^6 TU/ study eye. Show less

All-cause mortality

Arm/Group Title	Cohort 1	Cohort 2	Cohort 3	Cohort 4	Cohort 5	Cohort 6	Cohort 7
	Affected/at Risk (%)	Affected/at Risk (%)	Affected/at Risk (%)	Affected/at Risk (%)	Affected/at Risk (%)	Affected/at Risk (%)	Affected/at Risk (%)
Total	0/4 (0.00%)	0/4 (0.00%)	0/4 (0.00%)	0/4 (0.00%)	0/6 (0.00%)	0/4 (0.00%)	0/1 (0.00%)

Serious adverse events

Arm/Group Title	Cohort 1	Cohort 2	Cohort 3	Cohort 4	Cohort 5	Cohort 6	Cohort 7
	Affected/at Risk (%)	Affected/at Risk (%)	Affected/at Risk (%)	Affected/at Risk (%)	Affected/at Risk (%)	Affected/at Risk (%)	Affected/at Risk (%)

ARM/Group Title	Cohort 1	Cohort 2	Cohort 3	Cohort 4	Cohort 5	Cohort 6	Cohort 7
	Affected/at Risk (%)	Affected/at Risk (%)	Affected/at Risk (%)	Affected/at Risk (%)	Affected/at Risk (%)	Affected/at Risk (%)	Affected/at Risk (%)
Total	1/4 (25.00%)	0/4 (0.00%)	0/4 (0.00%)	0/4 (0.00%)	0/6 (0.00%)	1/4 (25.00%)	1/1 (100.00%)
Eye disorders							
Chorioretinopathy[a,b]	0/4 (0.00%)	0/4 (0.00%)	0/4 (0.00%)	0/4 (0.00%)	0/6 (0.00%)	0/4 (0.00%)	1/1 (100.00%)
Uveitis[a,b]	0/4 (0.00%)	0/4 (0.00%)	0/4 (0.00%)	0/4 (0.00%)	0/6 (0.00%)	1/4 (25.00%)	0/1 (0.00%)
Investigations							
Intraocular pressure increased[a,b]	1/4 (25.00%)	0/4 (0.00%)	0/4 (0.00%)	0/4 (0.00%)	0/6 (0.00%)	0/4 (0.00%)	0/1 (0.00%)
Other (Not Including Serious) Adverse Events							

0% Frequency threshold for reporting other adverse events

Arm/Group Title	Cohort 1	Cohort 2	Cohort 3	Cohort 4	Cohort 5	Cohort 6	Cohort 7
	Affected/at Risk (%)	Affected/at Risk (%)	Affected/at Risk (%)	Affected/at Risk (%)	Affected/at Risk (%)	Affected/at Risk (%)	Affected/at Risk (%)
Total	4/4 (100.00%)	4/4 (100.00%)	4/4 (100.00%)	4/4 (100.00%)	6/6 (100.00%)	4/4 (100.00%)	1/1 (100.00%)
Blood and lymphatic system disorders							
Lymphopenia[a,b]	0/4 (0.00%)	0/4 (0.00%)	0/4 (0.00%)	0/4 (0.00%)	0/6 (0.00%)	0/4 (0.00%)	0/1 (0.00%)
Cardiac disorders							
Ventricular extrasystoles[a,b]	0/4 (0.00%)	0/4 (0.00%)	0/4 (0.00%)	0/4 (0.00%)	0/6 (0.00%)	1/4 (25.00%)	0/1 (0.00%)
Eye disorders							
Anterior chamber cell[a,b]	0/4 (0.00%)	1/4 (25.00%)	0/4 (0.00%)	1/4 (25.00%)	0/6 (0.00%)	0/4 (0.00%)	0/1 (0.00%)
Anterior chamber inflammation[a,b]	0/4 (0.00%)	0/4 (0.00%)	0/4 (0.00%)	1/4 (25.00%)	0/6 (0.00%)	0/4 (0.00%)	0/1 (0.00%)
Cataract[a,b]	0/4 (0.00%)	1/4 (25.00%)	0/4 (0.00%)	0/4 (0.00%)	0/6 (0.00%)	0/4 (0.00%)	1/1 (100.00%)
Chalazion[a,b]	0/4 (0.00%)	0/4 (0.00%)	0/4 (0.00%)	0/4 (0.00%)	0/6 (0.00%)	1/4 (25.00%)	0/1 (0.00%)
Choroidal effusion[a,b]	0/4 (0.00%)	0/4 (0.00%)	0/4 (0.00%)	0/4 (0.00%)	1/6 (16.67%)	0/4 (0.00%)	0/1 (0.00%)

ARM/Group Title	Cohort 1	Cohort 2	Cohort 3	Cohort 4	Cohort 5	Cohort 6	Cohort 7
Conjunctival hemorrhage[a,b]	3/4 (75.00%)	2/4 (50.00%)	2/4 (50.00%)	1/4 (25.00%)	3/6 (50.00%)	0/4 (0.00%)	0/1 (0.00%)
Corneal disorder[a,b]	0/4 (0.00%)	1/4 (25.00%)	0/4 (0.00%)	0/4 (0.00%)	0/6 (0.00%)	0/4 (0.00%)	0/1 (0.00%)
Diplopia[a,b]	0/4 (0.00%)	0/4 (0.00%)	0/4 (0.00%)	0/4 (0.00%)	1/6 (16.67%)	0/4 (0.00%)	0/1 (0.00%)
Dyschromatopsia[a,b]	0/4 (0.00%)	0/4 (0.00%)	0/4 (0.00%)	0/4 (0.00%)	1/6 (16.67%)	0/4 (0.00%)	0/1 (0.00%)
Eye discharge[a,b]	1/4 (25.00%)	0/4 (0.00%)	0/4 (0.00%)	0/4 (0.00%)	0/6 (0.00%)	0/4 (0.00%)	0/1 (0.00%)
Eye disorder[a,b]	0/4 (0.00%)	0/4 (0.00%)	0/4 (0.00%)	0/4 (0.00%)	0/6 (0.00%)	1/4 (25.00%)	0/1 (0.00%)
Eye inflammation[a,b]	0/4 (0.00%)	0/4 (0.00%)	0/4 (0.00%)	0/4 (0.00%)	1/6 (16.67%)	0/4 (0.00%)	0/1 (0.00%)
Eye irritation[a,b]	0/4 (0.00%)	0/4 (0.00%)	0/4 (0.00%)	1/4 (25.00%)	2/6 (33.33%)	0/4 (0.00%)	0/1 (0.00%)
Eye pain[a,b]	2/4 (50.00%)	2/4 (50.00%)	1/4 (25.00%)	0/4 (0.00%)	1/6 (16.67%)	0/4 (0.00%)	1/1 (100.00%)
Eye pruritus[a,b]	0/4 (0.00%)	1/4 (25.00%)	2/4 (50.00%)	0/4 (0.00%)	2/6 (33.33%)	0/4 (0.00%)	0/1 (0.00%)
Eyelid irritation[a,b]	0/4 (0.00%)	0/4 (0.00%)	0/4 (0.00%)	0/4 (0.00%)	1/6 (16.67%)	0/4 (0.00%)	0/1 (0.00%)
Hypotony of eye[a,b]	0/4 (0.00%)	0/4 (0.00%)	0/4 (0.00%)	0/4 (0.00%)	0/6 (0.00%)	2/4 (50.00%)	0/1 (0.00%)
Keratic precipitates[a,b]	0/4 (0.00%)	0/4 (0.00%)	0/4 (0.00%)	1/4 (25.00%)	0/6 (0.00%)	0/4 (0.00%)	0/1 (0.00%)
Macular fibrosis[a,b]	0/4 (0.00%)	0/4 (0.00%)	0/4 (0.00%)	0/4 (0.00%)	1/6 (16.67%)	1/4 (25.00%)	0/1 (0.00%)
Macular oedema[a,b]	0/4 (0.00%)	0/4 (0.00%)	0/4 (0.00%)	0/4 (0.00%)	2/6 (33.33%)	0/4 (0.00%)	0/1 (0.00%)
Necrotizing retinitis[a,b]	0/4 (0.00%)	0/4 (0.00%)	0/4 (0.00%)	0/4 (0.00%)	0/6 (0.00%)	1/4 (25.00%)	0/1 (0.00%)
Ocular hyperemia[a,b]	1/4 (25.00%)	0/4 (0.00%)	0/4 (0.00%)	0/4 (0.00%)	0/6 (0.00%)	0/4 (0.00%)	0/1 (0.00%)
Ocular hypertension[a,b]	0/4 (0.00%)	0/4 (0.00%)	0/4 (0.00%)	0/4 (0.00%)	0/6 (0.00%)	0/4 (0.00%)	1/1 (100.00%)
Photopsia[a,b]	0/4 (0.00%)	0/4 (0.00%)	1/4 (25.00%)	0/4 (0.00%)	0/6 (0.00%)	1/4 (25.00%)	0/1 (0.00%)
Retinal disorder[a,b]	0/4 (0.00%)	0/4 (0.00%)	0/4 (0.00%)	0/4 (0.00%)	1/6 (16.67%)	0/4 (0.00%)	0/1 (0.00%)
Retinal hemorrhage[a,b]	0/4 (0.00%)	1/4 (25.00%)	0/4 (0.00%)	1/4 (25.00%)	1/6 (16.67%)	2/4 (50.00%)	0/1 (0.00%)

ARM/Group Title	Cohort 1	Cohort 2	Cohort 3	Cohort 4	Cohort 5	Cohort 6	Cohort 7
Retinal tear[a,b]	0/4 (0.00%)	0/4 (0.00%)	0/4 (0.00%)	0/4 (0.00%)	0/6 (0.00%)	1/4 (25.00%)	0/1 (0.00%)
Serous retinal detachment[a,b]	0/4 (0.00%)	0/4 (0.00%)	1/4 (25.00%)	0/4 (0.00%)	0/6 (0.00%)	0/4 (0.00%)	0/1 (0.00%)
Subretinal fibrosis[a,b]	0/4 (0.00%)	0/4 (0.00%)	0/4 (0.00%)	0/4 (0.00%)	0/6 (0.00%)	1/4 (25.00%)	0/1 (0.00%)
Subretinal fluid[a,b]	1/4 (25.00%)	1/4 (25.00%)	1/4 (25.00%)	0/4 (0.00%)	2/6 (33.33%)	0/4 (0.00%)	0/1 (0.00%)
Trichiasis[a,b]	1/4 (25.00%)	0/4 (0.00%)	0/4 (0.00%)	0/4 (0.00%)	0/6 (0.00%)	0/4 (0.00%)	0/1 (0.00%)
Uveitis[a,b]	0/4 (0.00%)	0/4 (0.00%)	0/4 (0.00%)	0/4 (0.00%)	0/6 (0.00%)	1/4 (25.00%)	0/1 (0.00%)
Vision blurred[a,b]	0/4 (0.00%)	0/4 (0.00%)	0/4 (0.00%)	0/4 (0.00%)	0/6 (0.00%)	0/4 (0.00%)	1/1 (100.00%)
Visual impairment[a,b]	0/4 (0.00%)	0/4 (0.00%)	0/4 (0.00%)	0/4 (0.00%)	1/6 (16.67%)	0/4 (0.00%)	1/1 (100.00%)
Vitreous detachment[a,b]	0/4 (0.00%)	0/4 (0.00%)	1/4 (25.00%)	0/4 (0.00%)	0/6 (0.00%)	0/4 (0.00%)	0/1 (0.00%)
Vitreous floaters[a,b]	1/4 (25.00%)	0/4 (0.00%)	1/4 (25.00%)	0/4 (0.00%)	2/6 (33.33%)	0/4 (0.00%)	0/1 (0.00%)
Vitreous hemorrhage[a,b]	0/4 (0.00%)	0/4 (0.00%)	0/4 (0.00%)	1/4 (25.00%)	0/6 (0.00%)	0/4 (0.00%)	0/1 (0.00%)
Xanthopsia[a,b]	0/4 (0.00%)	0/4 (0.00%)	0/4 (0.00%)	0/4 (0.00%)	1/6 (16.67%)	0/4 (0.00%)	0/1 (0.00%)
Gastrointestinal disorders							
Dental caries[a,b]	0/4 (0.00%)	0/4 (0.00%)	0/4 (0.00%)	0/4 (0.00%)	1/6 (16.67%)	0/4 (0.00%)	0/1 (0.00%)
Irritable bowel syndrome[a,b]	0/4 (0.00%)	1/4 (25.00%)	0/4 (0.00%)	0/4 (0.00%)	0/6 (0.00%)	0/4 (0.00%)	0/1 (0.00%)
Nausea[a,b]	0/4 (0.00%)	1/4 (25.00%)	0/4 (0.00%)	0/4 (0.00%)	1/6 (16.67%)	1/4 (25.00%)	1/1 (100.00%)
Vomiting[a,b]	0/4 (0.00%)	1/4 (25.00%)	0/4 (0.00%)	0/4 (0.00%)	0/6 (0.00%)	1/4 (25.00%)	0/1 (0.00%)
General disorders							
Asthenia[a,b]	0/4 (0.00%)	0/4 (0.00%)	1/4 (25.00%)	0/4 (0.00%)	0/6 (0.00%)	0/4 (0.00%)	0/1 (0.00%)
Influenza-like illness[a,b]	0/4 (0.00%)	0/4 (0.00%)	0/4 (0.00%)	0/4 (0.00%)	1/6 (16.67%)	0/4 (0.00%)	0/1 (0.00%)
Pain[a,b]	0/4 (0.00%)	0/4 (0.00%)	0/4 (0.00%)	0/4 (0.00%)	1/6 (16.67%)	0/4 (0.00%)	0/1 (0.00%)

ARM/Group Title	Cohort 1	Cohort 2	Cohort 3	Cohort 4	Cohort 5	Cohort 6	Cohort 7
Infections and infestations							
Conjunctivitis[a,b]	1/4 (25.00%)	1/4 (25.00%)	0/4 (0.00%)	0/4 (0.00%)	0/6 (0.00%)	0/4 (0.00%)	0/1 (0.00%)
Conjunctivitis viral[a,b]	1/4 (25.00%)	0/4 (0.00%)	0/4 (0.00%)	0/4 (0.00%)	0/6 (0.00%)	0/4 (0.00%)	0/1 (0.00%)
Diarrhoea infectious[a,b]	0/4 (0.00%)	1/4 (25.00%)	0/4 (0.00%)	0/4 (0.00%)	0/6 (0.00%)	0/4 (0.00%)	0/1 (0.00%)
Ear infection[a,b]	0/4 (0.00%)	1/4 (25.00%)	0/4 (0.00%)	0/4 (0.00%)	0/6 (0.00%)	0/4 (0.00%)	0/1 (0.00%)
Nasopharyngitis[a,b]	2/4 (50.00%)	2/4 (50.00%)	1/4 (25.00%)	0/4 (0.00%)	1/6 (16.67%)	0/4 (0.00%)	1/1 (100.00%)
Sinusitis[a,b]	0/4 (0.00%)	1/4 (25.00%)	0/4 (0.00%)	0/4 (0.00%)	0/6 (0.00%)	1/4 (25.00%)	0/1 (0.00%)
Injury, poisoning, and procedural complications							
Cartilage injury[a,b]	0/4 (0.00%)	0/4 (0.00%)	0/4 (0.00%)	0/4 (0.00%)	0/6 (0.00%)	0/4 (0.00%)	1/1 (100.00%)
Corneal abrasion[a,b]	1/4 (25.00%)	0/4 (0.00%)	0/4 (0.00%)	0/4 (0.00%)	0/6 (0.00%)	0/4 (0.00%)	0/1 (0.00%)
Tongue injury[a,b]	0/4 (0.00%)	1/4 (25.00%)	0/4 (0.00%)	0/4 (0.00%)	0/6 (0.00%)	0/4 (0.00%)	0/1 (0.00%)
Investigations							
Color vision tests abnormal[a,b]	0/4 (0.00%)	0/4 (0.00%)	0/4 (0.00%)	0/4 (0.00%)	0/6 (0.00%)	0/4 (0.00%)	1/1 (100.00%)
Fundoscopy abnormal[a,b]	0/4 (0.00%)	0/4 (0.00%)	0/4 (0.00%)	0/4 (0.00%)	1/6 (16.67%)	0/4 (0.00%)	0/1 (0.00%)
Intraocular pressure decreased[a,b]	0/4 (0.00%)	1/4 (25.00%)	0/4 (0.00%)	1/4 (25.00%)	2/6 (33.33%)	0/4 (0.00%)	0/1 (0.00%)
Intraocular pressure increased[a,b]	2/4 (50.00%)	3/4 (75.00%)	2/4 (50.00%)	1/4 (25.00%)	0/6 (0.00%)	0/4 (0.00%)	1/1 (100.00%)
Monoclonal immunoglobulin present[a,b]	0/4 (0.00%)	0/4 (0.00%)	0/4 (0.00%)	1/4 (25.00%)	0/6 (0.00%)	0/4 (0.00%)	0/1 (0.00%)
Visual field tests abnormal[a,b]	0/4 (0.00%)	0/4 (0.00%)	0/4 (0.00%)	0/4 (0.00%)	0/6 (0.00%)	1/4 (25.00%)	0/1 (0.00%)

ARM/Group Title	Cohort 1	Cohort 2	Cohort 3	Cohort 4	Cohort 5	Cohort 6	Cohort 7
Metabolism and nutrition disorders							
Decreased appetite[a,b]	0/4 (0.00%)	0/4 (0.00%)	0/4 (0.00%)	0/4 (0.00%)	0/6 (0.00%)	0/4 (0.00%)	1/1 (100.00%)
Musculoskeletal and connective tissue disorders							
Arthralgia[a,b]	0/4 (0.00%)	0/4 (0.00%)	0/4 (0.00%)	1/4 (25.00%)	0/6 (0.00%)	0/4 (0.00%)	0/1 (0.00%)
Arthritis[a,b]	0/4 (0.00%)	0/4 (0.00%)	0/4 (0.00%)	1/4 (25.00%)	0/6 (0.00%)	0/4 (0.00%)	0/1 (0.00%)
Back pain[a,b]	0/4 (0.00%)	0/4 (0.00%)	0/4 (0.00%)	0/4 (0.00%)	0/6 (0.00%)	0/4 (0.00%)	1/1 (100.00%)
Muscle spasms[a,b]	0/4 (0.00%)	1/4 (25.00%)	0/4 (0.00%)	0/4 (0.00%)	0/6 (0.00%)	0/4 (0.00%)	0/1 (0.00%)
Neck pain[a,b]	0/4 (0.00%)	0/4 (0.00%)	0/4 (0.00%)	0/4 (0.00%)	1/6 (16.67%)	0/4 (0.00%)	0/1 (0.00%)
Osteoarthritis[a,b]	0/4 (0.00%)	0/4 (0.00%)	0/4 (0.00%)	0/4 (0.00%)	1/6 (16.67%)	0/4 (0.00%)	0/1 (0.00%)
Pain in extremity[a,b]	0/4 (0.00%)	0/4 (0.00%)	0/4 (0.00%)	0/4 (0.00%)	0/6 (0.00%)	0/4 (0.00%)	1/1 (100.00%)
Synovial cyst[a,b]	0/4 (0.00%)	0/4 (0.00%)	0/4 (0.00%)	0/4 (0.00%)	1/6 (16.67%)	0/4 (0.00%)	0/1 (0.00%)
Nervous system disorders							
Dizziness[a,b]	0/4 (0.00%)	0/4 (0.00%)	0/4 (0.00%)	0/4 (0.00%)	0/6 (0.00%)	0/4 (0.00%)	1/1 (100.00%)
Headache[a,b]	1/4 (25.00%)	1/4 (25.00%)	0/4 (0.00%)	1/4 (25.00%)	1/6 (16.67%)	2/4 (50.00%)	1/1 (100.00%)
Tremor[a,b]	0/4 (0.00%)	0/4 (0.00%)	0/4 (0.00%)	0/4 (0.00%)	0/6 (0.00%)	0/4 (0.00%)	1/1 (100.00%)
Visual field defect[a,b]	0/4 (0.00%)	0/4 (0.00%)	0/4 (0.00%)	0/4 (0.00%)	1/6 (16.67%)	0/4 (0.00%)	0/1 (0.00%)
Psychiatric disorders							
Depression[a,b]	0/4 (0.00%)	0/4 (0.00%)	1/4 (25.00%)	0/4 (0.00%)	0/6 (0.00%)	0/4 (0.00%)	0/1 (0.00%)
Insomnia[a,b]	0/4 (0.00%)	1/4 (25.00%)	0/4 (0.00%)	0/4 (0.00%)	0/6 (0.00%)	0/4 (0.00%)	1/1 (100.00%)
Renal and urinary disorders							
Glycosuria[a,b]	0/4 (0.00%)	0/4 (0.00%)	0/4 (0.00%)	0/4 (0.00%)	1/6 (16.67%)	0/4 (0.00%)	0/1 (0.00%)
Leukocyturia[a,b]	0/4 (0.00%)	0/4 (0.00%)	0/4 (0.00%)	0/4 (0.00%)	1/6 (16.67%)	0/4 (0.00%)	0/1 (0.00%)
Respiratory, thoracic, and mediastinal disorders							
Cough[a,b]	0/4 (0.00%)	1/4 (25.00%)	0/4 (0.00%)	1/4 (25.00%)	0/6 (0.00%)	0/4 (0.00%)	1/1 (100.00%)
Oropharyngeal pain[a,b]	0/4 (0.00%)	1/4 (25.00%)	1/4 (25.00%)	0/4 (0.00%)	0/6 (0.00%)	0/4 (0.00%)	1/1 (100.00%)
Rhinorrhoea[a,b]	0/4 (0.00%)	0/4 (0.00%)	0/4 (0.00%)	0/4 (0.00%)	1/6 (16.67%)	0/4 (0.00%)	0/1 (0.00%)

ARM/Group Title	Cohort 1	Cohort 2	Cohort 3	Cohort 4	Cohort 5	Cohort 6	Cohort 7
Skin and subcutaneous tissue disorders							
Dermal cyst[a,b]	0/4 (0.00%)	0/4 (0.00%)	1/4 (25.00%)	0/4 (0.00%)	0/6 (0.00%)	0/4 (0.00%)	0/1 (0.00%)
Rash[a,b]	0/4 (0.00%)	0/4 (0.00%)	0/4 (0.00%)	0/4 (0.00%)	0/6 (0.00%)	1/4 (25.00%)	0/1 (0.00%)
Rash erythematous[a,b]	0/4 (0.00%)	0/4 (0.00%)	0/4 (0.00%)	0/4 (0.00%)	0/6 (0.00%)	1/4 (25.00%)	0/1 (0.00%)
Vascular disorders							
Hypertension[a,b]	0/4 (0.00%)	0/4 (0.00%)	0/4 (0.00%)	1/4 (25.00%)	0/6 (0.00%)	0/4 (0.00%)	0/1 (0.00%)

[a]Indicates events were collected by systematic assessment

[b]Term from vocabulary, MedDRA 22.1

United States

Terminated

Reason: Flavoprotein fluorescence machine for the trial is not working, so the trial was terminated. No study data were collected prior to termination.

Novel Quantification Methods for Fluorescence to Detect Progression in Stargardt Disease

ClinicalTrials.gov ID NCT01676766

Sponsor University of Michigan
Information provided by K. Thiran Jayasundera, University of Michigan (Responsible Party)
Last Update Posted 2016-11-08

Study Overview

Brief Summary
The purpose of this study is to utilize flavoprotein fluorescence and fundus autofluorescence to detect progression of Stargardt macular dystrophy in a pediatric population over the course of a year with the hope of aiding future therapeutic risk-benefit decisions and assessment of outcomes.

Stargardt macular dystrophy is the most common of the juvenile-onset macular dystrophies. Despite determination of ABCA4 as the causative gene, clinicians have been challenged by variability in clinical phenotypes. Given the recent initiation of clinical trials to assess novel treatments (e.g., gene therapy), there is a need to identify patients with the worst prognosis.

The investigators have observed that pediatric patients lose central visual function faster than their adult counterparts. Thus, they present an ideal cohort with which to determine the utility of novel modalities to detect early change. These include flavoprotein fluorescence, a new imaging technique for detecting mitochondrial dysfunction developed at the University of Michigan.

Fundus autofluorescence (FAF) is another commonly utilized technique of evaluating hereditary eye diseases. The investigators have developed a novel means of quantifying FAF signatures that will allow documentation of severity as well as detection of progression.

Detailed Description
This study will evaluate whether more sophisticated testing and analytic methodologies, including fundus autofluorescence (FAF) and a novel noninvasive method to measure retinal flavoprotein fluorescence (FPF), may be used to better predict Stargardt macular dystrophy progression and monitor treatment effects than

conventional modalities such as visual acuity and visual field. This method involves the use of novel statistical methods to assess the heterogeneity of fundus autofluorescence images.

Participants will complete 3 visits to the University of Michigan Kellogg Eye Center. Each visit will take approximately 2.5 hours. The initial visit will include a routine clinical eye examination, measurement of best-corrected visual acuity, indirect ophthalmoscopy, microperimetry, frequency-domain optical coherence tomography, Goldmann visual fields, fundus flavoprotein fluorescence (FPF) imaging, and fundus autofluorescence (FAF) and fundus photography. Patients will return for evaluation at 6 and 12 months after their initial visit to repeat testing and imaging.

Official Title

Novel Quantification Methods for Fundus Flavoprotein Fluorescence and Lipofuscin
  Fluorescence to Detect Progression in Stargardt Disease

Conditions

Stargardt Disease

Intervention/Treatment

Other Study ID Numbers

- HUM 64388

Study Start

2012-09

Primary Completion (Actual)

2016-10

Study Completion (Actual)

2016-10

Enrollment (Actual)

2

Study Type

Observational

United States
Michigan Locations

Ann Arbor, Michigan, United States, 48105
Kellogg Eye Center

Eligibility Criteria
Description

Inclusion Criteria

- Between the age of 5 and 18 years old
- Clinical diagnosis of Stargardt Disease

- Molecular confirmation of Stargardt Disease (with 2 identified mutations in ABCA4)
- Visual acuity better than 20/100

Exclusion Criteria
- Limited central vision, defined as visual acuity worse than 20/100
- A diagnosis of any other retinal degenerative disease

Study Population
We will perform an observational clinical study of 25 pediatric patients with Stargardt Disease recruited from the retinal degeneration clinic at the University of Michigan who have two mutations in ABCA4.

Ages Eligible for Study
5–18 Years (Child, Adult)

Sexes Eligible for Study
All

Accepts Healthy Volunteers
No
Sampling Method
Non-Probability Sample

Design Details
Observational Model: Case-Only
Time Perspective: Prospective
What is the study measuring?

Primary outcome measures

Outcome measure	Measure description	Time frame
Change from baseline in pixel intensity quantification of fundus autofluorescence at 6 months		0 months, 6 months
Change from baseline in pixel intensity quantification of flavoprotein autofluorescence at 6 months		0 months, 6 months

Secondary outcome measures

Outcome measure	Measure description	Time frame
Change from baseline in pixel intensity quantification of fundus autofluorescence at 12 months		0 months, 12 months
Change from baseline in pixel intensity quantification of flavoprotein autofluorescence at 12 months		0 months, 12 months

Collaborators and Investigators
This is where you will find people and organizations involved with this study.

Sponsor
University of Michigan

Collaborators
- Midwest Eye Banks

Investigators
- Principal Investigator: K. Thiran Jayasundera, MD, University of Michigan Kellogg Eye Center

General Publications
- Elner SG, Elner VM, Field MG, Park S, Heckenlively JR, Petty HR. Retinal flavoprotein autofluorescence as a measure of retinal health. Trans Am Ophthalmol Soc. 2008;106:215–22; discussion 222–4.
- Field MG, Elner VM, Park S, Hackel R, Heckenlively JR, Elner SG, Petty HR. Detection of retinal metabolic stress resulting from central serous retinopathy. Retina. 2009 Sep;29(8):1162-6. https://doi.org/10.1097/IAE.0b013e3181a3b923.
- Field MG, Elner VM, Puro DG, Feuerman JM, Musch DC, Pop-Busui R, Hackel R, Heckenlively JR, Petty HR. Rapid, noninvasive detection of diabetes-induced retinal metabolic stress. Arch Ophthalmol. 2008 Jul;126(7):934-8. https://doi.org/10.1001/archopht.126.7.934.
- Chen B, Tosha C, Gorin MB, Nusinowitz S. Analysis of autofluorescent retinal images and measurement of atrophic lesion growth in Stargardt disease. Exp Eye Res. 2010 Aug;91(2):143-52. https://doi.org/10.1016/j.exer.2010.03.021. Epub 2010 Apr 14.

United States

Terminated

Reason: There was no significant difference in our outcome measures between patients with disease versus controls, suggesting that our hypothesis is not substantiated. Since this was the major objective of the study, we decided to terminate the study.

Oxidative Stress in Stargardt Disease, Age-Related Macular Degeneration, and Diabetic Retinopathy

ClinicalTrials.gov ID NCT02875704

Sponsor Johns Hopkins University
Information provided by Johns Hopkins University (Responsible Party)
Last Update Posted 2022-09-26

Study Overview

Brief Summary
In this study, markers of oxidative stress will be measured in the aqueous humor of Stargardt disease, age-related macular degeneration, and diabetic retinopathy patients compared to controls.

Detailed Description
People with Stargardt disease, age-related macular degeneration (AMD), and diabetic retinopathy (DR) have decrease in central vision from damage to photoreceptors. One of the mechanisms causing damage is high levels of oxygen in the eye. This damage produces specific biomarkers that can be measured in eye fluid (aqueous humor). In this study, these biomarkers will be assessed in people with Stargardt disease, age-related macular degeneration, and diabetic retinopathy, compared to controls.

Official Title
Oxidative Stress in Stargardt Disease, Age-Related Macular Degeneration, and Diabetic Retinopathy

Conditions
Stargardt Disease
Diabetic Retinopathy
Macular Degeneration (Age Related)

Intervention/Treatment
- Other: Anterior Chamber (AC) Tap

Other Study ID Numbers
- IRB00112564
- OXI-SAD (Other Identifier) (OTHER: Other)

Study Start (Actual)
2017-01-03

Primary Completion (Actual)
2022-06-06

Study Completion (Actual)
2022-09-22

Enrollment (Actual)
77

Study Type
Observational

United States
Maryland Locations

Baltimore, Maryland, United States, 21287
Wilmer Eye Institute

Eligibility Criteria
Description

Inclusion Criteria
- Signed informed consent and authorization of use and disclosure of protected health information
- Age at least 18 years
- For the study group, patients diagnosed with Stargardt disease, age-related macular degeneration, and diabetic retinopathy by the investigators, based on clinical phenotype
- For the control group, patients with no retinal disease undergoing cataract surgery will be eligible.

Exclusion Criteria
- None

Study Population
Stargardt disease, AMD, DR patients, and controls

Ages Eligible for Study
18–100 Years (Adult, Older Adult)

Sexes Eligible for Study
All

Accepts Healthy Volunteers
No
Sampling Method
Non-Probability Sample

Design Details
Observational Model: Case-Control
Time Perspective: Prospective
Biospecimen Retention: Samples Without DNA
Biospecimen Description: Samples will only be used for measurement of biomarkers of oxidative stress

Cohorts and interventions

Group/cohort	Intervention/treatment
Stargardt disease, AMD, DR patients Stargardt disease, age-related macular degeneration, diabetic retinopathy patients	Other: Anterior Chamber (AC) Tap • Aqueous Samples will be collected for measurement of biomarkers • Other Names: – AC Tap
Controls Patients without retinal disease who will be undergoing cataract surgery	Other: Anterior Chamber (AC) Tap • Aqueous samples will be collected for measurement of biomarkers • Other Names: – AC Tap

Primary outcome measures

Outcome measure	Measure description	Time frame
Aqueous levels of oxidized adducts on protein (i.e., oxidative biomarker) in patients with Stargardt disease, AMD, DR, and controls	Baseline = Day of clinic visit for Stargardt disease, AMD, DR patients, and day of surgery for patients undergoing cataract surgery. No follow-up is required.	Baseline

Sponsor
Johns Hopkins University

Collaborators
No information provided

Investigators
• Principal Investigator: Peter A Campochiaro, MD, Johns Hopkins University

General Publications
No publications available

Chapter 8
Unknown Status Studies

China

Clinical Study of Subretinal Transplantation of Human Embryo Stem Cell-Derived Retinal Pigment Epitheliums in Treatment of Macular Degeneration Diseases

ClinicalTrials.gov ID NCT02749734

Sponsor Southwest Hospital, China
Information provided by Zheng Qin Yin, Southwest Hospital, China
(Responsible Party)
Last Update Posted 2018-01-31

Study Overview

Brief Summary
The purpose of this study is to determine the safety and therapeutic effect of subretinal transplantation of human embryo stem cell-derived retinal pigment epitheliums (hESC-RPE) in patients with macular degeneration diseases and explore new treatment modalities for macular degeneration diseases (Age-related macular degeneration and Stargardt's macular dystrophy).

Official Title
Clinical Study of Subretinal Transplantation of Human Embryo Stem Cell-Derived Retinal Pigment Epitheliums in Treatment of Macular Degeneration Diseases

Conditions
Macular Degeneration
Stargardt's Macular Dystrophy

© The Author(s), under exclusive license to Springer Nature Switzerland AG 2024

J. N. Weiss, *Clinical Trials in Stargardt Disease Treatment*, https://doi.org/10.1007/978-3-031-58807-5_8

Intervention/Treatment
- Procedure: Subretinal transplantation

Other Study ID Numbers
- 2013CB967002

Study Start
2015-05

Primary Completion (Estimated)
2018-12

Study Completion (Estimated)
2019-12

Enrollment (Estimated)
15

Study Type
Interventional

Phase
Phase 1 and Phase 2

China
Chongqing Locations

Chongqing, Chongqing, China, 400038
Southwest Hospital

Eligibility Criteria
Description

Inclusion Criteria
- Aging from 18 to 75 years
- Must have signed informed consent
- At least one visually impaired eye caused by macular degeneration diseases
- Cannot be effectively treated with conventional therapies
- Best-corrected visual acuity scores between 19 and 73 letter in ETDRs (early treatment diabetic retinopathy) eye chart, including 19 and 73 (or the equivalent of Snellen eyesight from 20/400 to 20/40)
- Visual loss caused by macular degeneration diseases

Exclusion Criteria
- Eyes with concomitant diseases which will interfere the visual improvement of the study
- Active intraocular inflammation regardless of the grade of severity
- Active infection (e.g., conjunctivitis, keratitis, scleritis, uveitis, ophthalmia)
- History of uveitis
- Severe cataract, glaucoma, retinal blood vessels occlusion, retinal detachment, macular hole, vitreous-macula traction

- Iris neovascularization
- Patients who have only one functioning eye, or the best-corrected vision of untreated eye scores less than 24 letters in ETDRS chart (corresponding to 20/320 in Snellen chart)
- History of intraocular surgery
- Severe systemic diseases: Stroke, coronary heart disease, angina pectoris, renal insufficiency needing dialysis
- Allergic to sodium fluorescein
- Uncontrolled hypertension (systolic pressure > 140 mmHg, or diastolic pressure > 90 mmHg)
- Coagulative function disorder
- System administration of drugs that are toxic to lens, retina, or optic nerve like hydroxychloroquine, phenothiazine, ethambutol, tamoxifen, etc.
- Involved in other clinical trials of any medicine within 1 month (or within 5 half-life periods)
- Have maternity plan in 6 months
- In pregnancy or lactation period.

Ages Eligible for Study
18–75 Years (Adult, Older Adult)

Sexes Eligible for Study
All

Accepts Healthy Volunteers
No

Design Details
Primary Purpose: Treatment
Allocation: N/A
Interventional Model: Single Group Assignment
Masking: None (Open Label)

Arms and interventions

Participant group/arm	Intervention/treatment
Experimental: hESC-RPE Subretinal transplantation of human embryo stem cell-derived retinal pigment epitheliums	Procedure: Subretinal transplantation • Transplant hESC-RPE into subretinal space of patients with macular degeneration

Primary outcome measures

Outcome measure	Measure description	Time frame
Number of participants with Treatment-Related Adverse Events [Safety and Tolerability]	Patients with Treatment-Related Adverse Events caused by local rejection of implanted cells or systemic immunosuppression treatment	Up to 12 months

Secondary outcome measures

Outcome measure	Measure description	Time frame
Number of Early Treatment Diabetic Retinopathy (ETDRS) letters participants can recognize	Visual acuity is reflected by number of ETDRS letters participants can recognize	Up to 12 months
Visual field as examined by static perimetry	Area and sensitivity of visual field are detected by static perimetry	Up to 12 months
Flash Electroretinogram (FERG)	Retinal electrophysiological function is tested by FERG	Up to 12 months
Amplitude and Latency of Flash Visual-Evoked Potentials (FVEP)	Optic nerve function as assessed by FVEP	Up to 12 months
Multifocal Electroretinogram (MFERG)	Local retinal function as assessed by MFERG	Up to 12 months

Sponsor
Southwest Hospital, China

Collaborators
No information provided

Investigators
No information provided

General Publications
No publications available

Europe

Unknown Status

Saffron Supplementation in Stargardt's Disease (STARSAF02)

ClinicalTrials.gov ID NCT01278277

Sponsor Catholic University of the Sacred Heart
Information provided by Benedetto Falsini, Catholic University of the Sacred Heart
(Responsible Party)
Last Update Posted 2017-07-19

Study Overview

Brief Summary
The general area of research in which this project has been designed is that of retinal degeneration related to mutations in the ABCR gene, responsible for Stargardt disease/fundus flavimaculatus retinal dystrophy (STD/FF). STG/FF is one of the major

causes of vision impairment in the young age. STG/FF originates typically from the dysfunction and loss of cone and rod photoreceptors, developing through a photo-oxidative mechanism. The major disease locus is the central retina, i.e., the macula, whose neurons have the highest density and underlie critical functions such as visual acuity, color vision, and contrast sensitivity. There is currently no cure for STG/FF. Recent experimental findings indicate that Saffron, derived from the pistils of Crocus Sativus, may have a role as a retinal neuro-protectant against oxidative damage. The stigmata of Crocus sativus contain biologically high concentrations of chemical compounds including crocin, crocetin, whose multiple C=C bonds provide the antioxidant potential. In addition, it is well known that this compound is safe and free of adverse side effects. The aim of this research is to investigate the influence of short-term Saffron supplementation on retinal function in STG/FF patients carrying ABCR mutations. The macular cone-mediated electroretinogram (ERG) in response to high-frequency flicker (focal flicker ERG) will be employed as the main outcome variable. Secondary outcome variable will be the psychophysical cone system recovery after bleaching.

Detailed Description

Research Plan Background: Stargardt disease (STGD/FFM) is the most common hereditary recessive macular dystrophy characterized by juvenile to young adult onset, central visual impairment, progressive bilateral atrophy of the macula, and retinal pigment epithelium (RPE), with a frequent appearance of orange/yellow flecks distributed around the macula and/or the mid-retinal periphery. A clinically similar retinal disorder, fundus flavimaculatus (FFM), often displays later ages of onset and slower progression. It has been suggested and demonstrated that STGD and FFM represent allelic disorders. Mutations in the gene encoding an ATP-binding cassette (ABC) transporter (ABCR), mapping to chromosome 1p13-p21, have been found to be responsible of STGD. The ABCR gene is expressed exclusively and at high levels in the retina, in both rod and cone photoreceptors. A recent study, investigating the molecular mechanisms underlying photoreceptor degeneration in ABCR knock-out mice, proposed that photoreceptors die as a consequence of 'poisoning' of the RPE by lipofuscin accumulation and loss of the RPE support role. Accumulation within the RPE cells of a compound, A2E, forming from condensation of phosphatydilethanlolamine and the all-trans-retinal released from photoactivated rhodopsin, probably leads in vivo to an increased absorption of blue lights and to phototoxic RPE cell damage. The mutation-induced disease may affect both rod and cone photoreceptors, at relatively early stages. In vitro studies also demonstrated that the ABCR itself is an efficient target of all-trans-retinal-mediated photooxidative damage.

Clinically, many reports have documented an abnormal functioning of both macular and peripheral cones, as well as rods, in STGD/FFM. There is also evidence that STGD/FFM may be associated with different patterns of retinal dysfunction, with a selective involvement of macular function, or more widespread dysfunction involving cone and/or rod function, showing intrafamilial consistency. Characteristic abnormalities of dark adaptation, involving a delayed post-bleach recovery, to the baseline sensitivity, of the last branch of the adaptation curve have been also described. Similar abnormalities in rod dark adaptation have been recently found in mice heterozygous for a null mutation in the ABCR gene. Clinical evidence indicates that the recovery of cone sensitivity after bleaching is also severely impaired in STG/FF, suggesting that profoundly altered retinoid recycling, leading to photooxidative damage, specifically occurs in cone photoreceptors.

Recent experimental findings indicate that Saffron, derived from the pistils of Crocus Sativus, may have a role as a retinal neuro-protectant against oxidative damage. Indeed, Saffron has been shown to be protective, for both morphology and function, in a rat model of light-induced photoreceptor degeneration. In this model, cell death is thought to result from oxidative stress induced by prolonged increase in oxygen tension and photooxidation. Saffron is an attractive candidate to be tested because the stigmata of Crocus sativus contain biologically high concentrations of interesting chemical compounds including crocin, crocetin, whose multiple $C=C$ bonds give the antioxidant potential. Not to mention that its centuries-long use as spice, with no known ill effects, increases the confidence in secure applicability. In addition, it has been recently reported that crocins are able to activate metabolic pathways to protect cells from apoptosis and to reduce light-induced death in isolated photoreceptors, while crocetin increases oxygen diffusivity through liquids, such as plasma. Considering the high metabolic rate of photoreceptors, the availability of oxygen may be a critical factor in protecting them from death.

Metabolites of antioxidant flavonoids bind directly to DNA and induce its partial conformation to beta-DNA, thereby protecting the cell from damage. Based on these observations, it comes clear that Saffron extract does not act as a simple antioxidant. The peculiar characteristics of Saffron components support the hypothesis of an involvement of very different ways of action going from antioxidant activity to direct control of gene expression. These components may act in humans as protective agents against oxidative damage for the aging retina and may repair early photoreceptor damage associated with STG/FF, whose disease pathophysiology has been linked by experimental studies to light-induced oxidative damage to the outer retina. In STG/FF eyes, at early disease stages, the normal number of cone photoreceptors is partially retained, although the cells might be dysfunctional. As a result of the rescuing effects of Saffron, the pool of damaged but viable photoreceptors could increase its response, resulting in improved retinal sensitivity.

The objective of the present project is to evaluate whether Saffron supplementation has a beneficial neuro-protective effect for the damaged retinas as a consequence of ABCR mutation-STD/FF.

Clinical Protocol Patients: A group of 30 STG/FF patients (14 males, 16 females, age range: 15–68 years) will be included in this study. Patients will meet the following inclusion criteria: (1) Macular and peripheral retinal degeneration with typical funduscopic lesions (retinal flecks) and a cone-rod pattern of retinal dysfunction, as determined by standard Ganzfeld electroretinography and dark-adapted fundus perimetry, and classic fundus appearance, (2) Relatively preserved central retinal function (visual field by Goldmann V/4e > 30°, corrected EDTRS visual acuity >20/80) and stable central fixation as determined by a Visuskope, (3) Known genotype or genotype under study, (4) At least four follow-up clinical examinations over the past 3 years, (5) No or minimal ocular media opacities, (6) No concomitant ocular (e.g., glaucoma, amblyopia) or systemic diseases. Informed consent for all patients and controls will be obtained after the aims and procedures of the study will be explained in detail.

Treatment and Testing Schedule: The patients will be divided into two groups: 15 will be treated with oral supplementation of a daily dose of Saffron for 90 days, and 15 will undergo placebo treatment during the same period. At the end of a 90 days period, the patients will be crossed over and assigned, respectively, to placebo or Saffron supplementation. In all patients, clinical examination, including visual acuity testing with a calibrated standard Snellen chart and fundus examination by direct and indirect ophthalmoscopy, and FERG testing will be performed at the study entry (baseline) and after 180 days of treatment or placebo. In all cases, compliance will be judged by telephone interview and pill counts. Adverse side effects will be reported.

Electrophysiological Methods: FERG testing will be performed according to a previously published technique. Briefly, ERGs will be elicited by the LED-generated sinusoidal luminance modulation of a circular uniform field (18° in diameter, 80 cd/m^2 mean luminance, dominant wavelength: 630 nm), presented at the frequency of 41 Hz on the rear of a ganzfeld bowl, illuminated at the same mean luminance as the stimulus. A series of FERG responses will be collected at different modulation depths [quantified by the Michelson luminance contrast formula: 100%*(Lmax -Lmin)/(Lmax +Lmin), where Lmax and Lmin are maximum and minimum luminance, respectively] between 16.5% and 93.8% in 0.1–0.3 log unit steps. FERG signals will be acquired in sequence for six values of modulation depth between 16.5% and 93.5%, presented in an increasing order. For each patient, FERG log amplitudes will be plotted as a function of log modulation depth. The resulting function's slope will be determined by a linear regression. From the same regression line, FERG threshold will be estimated from the value of log modulation depth yielding a criterion amplitude, corresponding to a S/N ratio of 3.

Psychophysics: An increment threshold technique will be used to evaluate the recovery of cone system sensitivity after bleaching exposure. Psychophysical threshold will be determined at the paracentral visual field locations with preserved visual sensitivity, by presenting a 0.5 s flashing light on a light adapting background of 20 cd/sqm. Following baseline assessment, the threshold intensity for the flashed light will be measured and plotted as a function of time, following a 30 s exposure to an adapting light (delivered in Maxwellian view by means of a calibrated indirect ophthalmoscope) whose intensity is estimated bleach approx 30% of the cone photopigment. The resulting dynamic recovery function, fitted by an exponential function, describes the sensitivity recovery of the photopic system following bleaching and reflects either the rate of free opsin inactivation or photopigment synthesis. A computer-controlled system, employing a commercially available apparatus, has been developed for measuring bleaching adaptation of the cone system.

Statistical Analysis: Sample size estimates of patients for this study will be based on previous investigations where the between- and within-subjects variability (expressed as data SD) of FERG parameters was determined in STG/FF patients. Assuming between- and within-subjects SDs in FERG amplitude and phase of 0.1 logmicroV and 20 degrees, respectively, the sample sizes of patients assigned to both Saffron and placebo provide a power of 80%, at an alpha = 0.05, for detecting in each group a test-retest difference (i.e., 90 days minus baseline test) of 0.1 logmicroV (SD: 0.1) and 30 degrees (SD: 20) in amplitude and phase, respectively. Results will be analyzed by multivariate statistics (multivariate analysis of variance for repeated measures, MANOVA). In all the analyses, a $p < 0.05$ will be considered as statistically significant.

Official Title

A Novel Therapeutic Strategy Targeting Photoreceptor Oxidative Damage in ABCR-Related Retinal Degenerations

Conditions

Retinal Degeneration
Genetic Disease
Single-Gene Defects
Macular Dystrophy

Intervention/Treatment

- Dietary Supplement: Saffron supplementation
- Other: placebo

Other Study ID Numbers

- STARSAF02

Study Start

2011-02

Primary Completion (Estimated)

2017-11

Study Completion (Estimated)

2017-12

Enrollment (Estimated)

30

Study Type

Interventional

Phase
Phase 1 and Phase 2

Italy

Rome, Italy, 00168
Policlinico A. Gemelli

Eligibility Criteria
Description

Inclusion Criteria
- Macular and peripheral retinal degeneration with typical funduscopic lesions (retinal flecks)
- Relatively preserved central retinal function
- Known genotype or genotype under study

Exclusion Criteria
- absence of a rod-cone pattern of dysfunction
- acuity less than 0.1
- Unknown genotype

Ages Eligible for Study
8–60 Years (Child, Adult)

Sexes Eligible for Study
All

Accepts Healthy Volunteers
No

Design Details
Primary Purpose: Treatment
Allocation: Randomized
Interventional Model: Crossover Assignment
Masking: Double (Participant Investigator)

Arms and interventions

Participant group/arm	Intervention/treatment
Placebo Comparator: placebo supplementation patients will be assigned, in a cross-over design, to placebo or supplement administration	Other: placebo • Placebo supplementation
Active Comparator: Saffron Saffron Supplementation 20 mg/die	Dietary Supplement: Saffron supplementation • Saffron supplementation 20 mg • Other Names: – Zaffit Special

Primary outcome measures

Outcome measure	Measure description	Time frame
Focal electroretinogram (FERG)	ERGs will be elicited by the LED-generated sinusoidal luminance modulation of a circular uniform field (18° in diameter, 80 cd/m² mean luminance, dominant wavelength: 630 nm), presented at the frequency of 41 Hz on the rear of a ganzfeld bowl, illuminated at the same mean luminance as the stimulus.	6 months

Secondary outcome measures

Outcome measure	Measure description	Time frame
Psychophysical recovery of cone system sensitivity after bleaching	Psychophysical threshold will be determined at the paracentral visual field locations with preserved visual sensitivity, by presenting a 0.5 s flashing light on a light adapting background of 20 cd/sqm. Following baseline assessment, the threshold intensity for the flashed light will be measured and plotted as a function of time, following 30 s exposure to an adapting light (delivered in Maxwellian view by means of a calibrated indirect ophthalmoscope) whose intensity is estimated bleach approx 30% of the cone photopigment.	6 months

Sponsor
Catholic University of the Sacred Heart

Collaborators
No information provided

Investigators
- Principal Investigator: Benedetto Falsini, MD, Catholic University of the Sacred Heart
- Principal Investigator: Marco Piccardi, MD, Catholic University of the Sacred Heart
- Study Director: Silvia Bisti, PhD, University of L'Aquila

General Publications
- Falsini B, Piccardi M, Minnella A, Savastano C, Capoluongo E, Fadda A, Balestrazzi E, Maccarone R, Bisti S. Influence of saffron supplementation on retinal flicker sensitivity in early age-related macular degeneration. Invest Ophthalmol Vis Sci. 2010 Dec;51(12):6118–24. https://doi.org/10.1167/iovs.09-4995. Epub 2010 Aug 4.

Europe

Unknown Status

Stem Cells Therapy in Degenerative Diseases of the Retina

ClinicalTrials.gov ID NCT03772938

Sponsor Pomeranian Medical University Szczecin
Information provided by Marta P. Wiącek, Pomeranian Medical University Szczecin
   (Responsible Party)
Last Update Posted 2018-12-17

Study Overview

Brief Summary

The purpose of this study is to test the safety and effectiveness of an autologous bone marrow-derived stem/progenitor cells administered intravitreously in the subjects with degenerative diseases of the retina.

Detailed Description

Degenerative diseases of the retina are challenging for ophthalmologists. This is a common term that covers heterogenous group of diseases, i.e., retinitis pigmentosa, Stargardt disease, Best's disease, or age-related macular degeneration. Undetermined etiology, wide range of factors that may trigger the onset of the disease and modulate its course, impedes the implementation of an effective treatment. Currently, a stem cells therapy seems to be promising option in patients with degenerative diseases of the retina. The purpose of this prospective, non-randomized, open label, pilot study is to conduct the investigation of the safety and efficacy of intravitreal injection of autologous bone marrow-isolated stem/progenitor cells with different selected phenotypes into the subjects with degenerative diseases of the retina. Especially, this clinical trial is designated to test the therapeutic (pro-regenerative and neuro-protective) functions of different stem/progenitor cell populations able to secrete bioactive neurotrophic factors. All patients enrolled will have a documented history of degenerative disease of the retina prior to study enrollment. Next, an intravitreous injection of autologous bone marrow-isolated stem/progenitor cells will be performed.

Finally, treatment safety, adverse events, and exploratory parameters, including best-corrected visual acuity, visual field, and electroretinography parameters, to establish disease progression rate will be recorded throughout the duration of the posttreatment follow-up period.

Official Title

Stem Cells Therapy in Degenerative Diseases of the Retina

Conditions
Retinal Degeneration
Retinitis Pigmentosa
Age-Related Macular Degeneration
Stargardt Disease 1

Intervention/Treatment
- Biological: Stem/progenitor cells transplantation

Other Study ID Numbers
- IKiKO-KB-0012/143/13

Study Start (Actual)
2018-12-13

Primary Completion (Estimated)
2020-02-28

Study Completion (Estimated)
2020-03-31

Enrollment (Estimated)
30

Study Type
Interventional

Phase
Phase 1

Poland

Szczecin, Poland, 70-111
I Department of Ophthalmology

Eligibility Criteria
Description

Inclusion Criteria
- diagnosed degenerative disease of the retina,
- age 18–65 years,
- best-corrected visual acuity max. 0,2 (Snellen letter chart),
- good understanding of the protocol and willingness to consent,
- signed informed consent.

Exclusion Criteria
- concomitant eye disease (glaucoma, etc.)
- concomitant of other systemic disease or diseases,
- inflammation (high protein or lymphocytosis in the CSF), active infections.
- diabetes,

- cardiovascular disorders,
- cancer,
- autoimmune diseases,
- renal failure,
- impaired hepatic function,
- subject unwilling or unable to comply with the requirements of the protocol,
- patient has been treated previously with any cellular therapy.

Ages Eligible for Study

18–65 Years (Adult, Older Adult)

Sexes Eligible for Study

All

Accepts Healthy Volunteers

No

Design Details

Primary Purpose: Other
Allocation: Non-Randomized
Interventional Model: Parallel Assignment
Masking: None (Open Label)

Arms and interventions

Participant group/arm	Intervention/treatment
Active Comparator: Stem/progenitor cells transplantation Intervention: A single intravitreal injection of autologous bone marrow-derived stem/progenitor cells will be performed.	Biological: Stem/progenitor cells transplantation • Human autologous bone marrow-derived stem/progenitor cell transplantation administered as an intravitreal injection in patients with degenerative disease of retina.
Sham Comparator: Standard treatment of degenerative disease of retina Symptomatic treatment of degenerative disease of retina without biologic cell-based treatment	Biological: Stem/progenitor cells transplantation • Human autologous bone marrow-derived stem/progenitor cell transplantation administered as an intravitreal injection in patients with degenerative disease of retina.

Primary outcome measures

Outcome measure	Measure description	Time frame
Number of participants with treatment-related adverse events as assessed by CTCAE v4.0	Confirm the safety of autologous bone marrow stem/progenitor cell intravitreal injection in enrolled patients by repeated follow-up over 1 year with clinical evaluations.	12 months

Secondary outcome measures

Outcome measure	Measure description	Time frame
Efficacy of autologous bone marrow stem/progenitor intravitreal injection in enrolled patients.	Best-corrected visual acuity, ETDRS chart [number of letters]	12 months
Intraocular pressure	Pascal tonometer [mmHg]	12 months
Optic disk retinal nerve fiber layer	Optical coherence tomography [um]	12 months
Central macular thickness	Optical coherence tomography [um]	12 months
Ganglion cell complex thickness	Optical coherence tomography [um]	12 months
Choroidal thickness	Enhanced depth imaging optical coherence tomography [um]	12 months
Choroidal volume	Enhanced depth imaging optical coherence tomography [mm^3]	12 months
Computed perimetry (30–2 and 10–2 module)	Mean deviation, pattern standard deviation [B]	12 months
Goldmann perimetry with color filters	[degrees]	12 months
Contrast sensitivity	Pelli-Robson chart [number of letters]	12 months
Function of the photoreceptors (rods and cones), inner retinal cells (bipolar and amacrine cells), and ganglion cells.	Electroretinography (ERG) examination: • Amplitude of a and b waves [V], • Culmination time of a and b waves [s], • Culmination time of q1-q3 waves [s].	12 months
Function of the photoreceptors	Multifocal electroretinography (mfERG) examination: • Retinal response density [V/degree 2], • Culmination time of P1 wave in 6 rings [s].	12 months
Function of ganglion cells	Pattern electroretinography (PERG) examination: • Amplitude of P50 and N95 waves [V], • Culmination time of P50 wave [s].	12 months

Sponsor

Pomeranian Medical University Szczecin

Collaborators

No information provided

Investigators

• Study Chair: Bogusław Machaliński, MD, PhD, Pomeranian Medical University
• Study Director: Anna Machalińska, MD, PhD, Pomeranian Medical University

General Publications

No publications available

Korea

Unknown Status

Safety and Tolerability of MA09-hRPE Cells in Patients with Stargardt's Macular Dystrophy (SMD)

ClinicalTrials.gov ID NCT01625559

Sponsor CHABiotech CO., Ltd.
Information provided by CHABiotech CO., Ltd. (Responsible Party)
Last Update Posted 2015-02-18

Study Overview

Brief Summary
The purpose of this study is:

- To evaluate the safety and tolerability of RPE cellular therapy in patients with SMD Group
- When-MA09-hRPE cell transplantation to evaluate the safety of surgical procedures.
- In future studies intended to assess the number of transplanted hRPE cells.
- In the past, MA09-hRPE cell therapy used in the study was to evaluate the validity of the potential.
- Homologous retinal pigment epithelial cells derived from embryonic stem cells, future studies of drugs that are used in representing the potential validity to evaluate the optimal dose.

Official Title
A Phase I, Open-Label, Prospective Study to Determine the Safety and Tolerability of Subretinal Transplantation of Human Embryonic Stem Cell-Derived Retinal Pigmented Epithelial (MA09-hRPE) Cells in Patients With Stargardt's Macular Dystrophy (SMD)

Conditions
Stargardt's Macular Dystrophy

Intervention/Treatment
- Biological: MA09-hRPE

Other Study ID Numbers
- CHA_CTP_0903

Study Start
2012-09

Primary Completion (Estimated)
2015-03

Study Completion (Estimated)
2015-06

Enrollment (Estimated)
3

Study Type
Interventional

Phase
Phase 1

Korea, Republic of
Gyeonggi-do Locations

Seongnam-si, Gyeonggi-do, Korea, Republic of, 463-712
CHA Bundang Medical Center

Eligibility Criteria
Description

Inclusion Criteria
* Adult male or female over 20 years of age.
* Clinical diagnosis of advanced SMD.
* The visual acuity of the eye to receive the transplant will be no better than hand movement.
* The visual acuity of the eye that is not to receive the transplant will be no better than 24 (20/320) Early Treatment of Diabetic Retinopathy Study (ETDRS) letters.

Exclusion Criteria
* History of malignancy.
* History of myocardial infarction in previous 12 months.
* History of diabetes mellitus.
* Any immunodeficiency.
* Any current immunosuppressive therapy other than intermittent or low-dose corticosteroids.
* Serologic evidence of infection with Hepatitis B, Hepatitis C, or HIV.
* Current participation in any other clinical trial.
* Participation within previous 6 months in any clinical trial of a drug by ocular or systemic administration.
* Any other sight-threatening ocular disease.
* Any chronic ocular medications. Any history of retinal vascular disease (compromised blood-retinal barrier). Glaucoma. Uveitis or other intraocular inflammatory disease. Significant lens opacities or other media opacity. Ocular lens removal within previous 3 months

Ages Eligible for Study
20 Years and older (Adult, Older Adult)

Sexes Eligible for Study
All

Accepts Healthy Volunteers
No

Design Details
Primary Purpose: Treatment
Allocation: N/A
Interventional Model: Single Group Assignment
Masking: None (Open Label)

Arms and interventions

Participant group/arm	Intervention/treatment
Experimental: 50,000 cells Biological: MA09-hRPE Cellular therapy	Biological: MA09-hRPE • MA09-hRPE: 50,000 cells

Primary outcome measures

Outcome measure	Measure description	Time frame
Safety and tolerance of transplantation	The transplantation of hESC-derived RPE cells MA09-hRPE will be considered safe and tolerated in the absence of: 1. Any grade 2 (NCI grading system) or greater adverse event related to the cell product 2. Any evidence that the cells are contaminated with an infectious agent 3. Any evidence that the cells show tumorigenic potential	18 months

Secondary outcome measures

Outcome measure	Measure description	Time frame
Evidence of successful engraftment	Evidence of successful engraftment. Evidence of successful engraftment will consist of: Structural evidence (OCT imaging, fluorescein angiography, autofluorescence photography, slit-lamp examination with fundus photography) that cells have been implanted in the correct location; Electroretinographic evidence (mfERG) showing enhanced activity in the implant location	18 months

Sponsor
CHABiotech CO., Ltd.

Collaborators
No information provided

Investigators
- Principal Investigator: Wonkyung Song, MD. PhD., CHA Bundang
  Medical Center

General Publications
No publications available

United Kingdom

Unknown Status

**Visual Performance Measures in a Virtual Reality Environment
for Assessing Clinical Trial Outcomes in Those with Severely
Reduced Vision**

ClinicalTrials.gov ID NCT04281732

Sponsor Queen's University, Belfast
Information provided by Ruth Hogg, Queen's University, Belfast (Responsible Party)
Last Update Posted 2020-02-24

Study Overview

Brief Summary

Purpose
To validate a newly developed battery of performance-based tests of visual function
to be presented using virtual reality. The tests are intended as potential outcome
measures for clinical trials of treatments of eye disease: they measure visual
performance in patients with low vision on visual tasks that are relevant for
daily life.

Detailed Description
Aims of the Research Project
1. To validate a new virtual reality (VR)-based battery of performance-based tests
   of visual function that are relevant for patients' daily lives.
2. To quantify the reproducibility of the performance-based tests.
3. To gather acceptability and ease-of-use data from patients.

Official Title
Visual Performance Measures in a Virtual Reality Environment for Assessing
Clinical Trial Outcomes in Those With Severely Reduced Vision

Conditions
Low Vision
Retinitis Pigmentosa
Stargardt Disease 1
Stargardt Disease 3
Stargardt Disease 4
Albinism
Show fewer conditions

Intervention/Treatment
- Device: Virtual Reality Headset-based tests

Other Study ID Numbers
- 17/NI/0002

Study Start (Actual)
2018-10-01

Primary Completion (Estimated)
2020-09-30

Study Completion (Estimated)
2020-12-31

Enrollment (Estimated)
20

Study Type
Observational

Study Contact
Name: Ruth Hogg, PhD
Phone Number: 02890971654
Email: r.e.hogg@qub.ac.uk
Study Contact Backup
Name: Lucie Dalton, BSc
Email: l.dalton@qub.ac.uk
United Kingdom
Northern Ireland Locations

Belfast, Northern Ireland, United Kingdom, BT9 7AB
Recruiting
NI Clinical Research Facility

Contact
Ruth Hogg
02890635018 r.e.hogg@qub.ac.uk

Eligibility Criteria
Description

Inclusion Criteria
- Male and female participants
- Age 20–50
- Bilateral sight impairment due to Stargardt's disease, retinitis pigmentosa, or albinism.
- Sight impairment criteria are as follows:

  - Visual acuity of 3/60 to 6/60 with a full field of vision.
  - Visual acuity of up to 6/24 with a moderate reduction of field of vision

Exclusion Criteria
- Any physical impairment that would make use of the virtual reality headset difficult or unsafe.
- A history of vertigo or dizziness.

Study Population
Patients with Stargardt's disease, advanced retinitis pigmentosa, and albinism.

Ages Eligible for Study
20–50 Years (Adult)

Sexes Eligible for Study
All
Sampling Method
Non-Probability Sample

Design Details
Observational Model: Cohort
Time Perspective: Prospective

Cohorts and interventions

Intervention/treatment
Device: Virtual Reality Headset-based tests • Visual task tests based on Oculus Rift

Primary outcome measures

Outcome measure	Measure description	Time frame
Test repeatability	Bland and Altman analysis will be used to investigate the repeatability of the tests between visit 1 and visit 2.	All statistical analyses will take place once all data collection has ended, average 1 year.

Secondary outcome measures

Outcome measure	Measure description	Time frame
Ease of use and acceptability questionnaire	Modified from Tay et al., Br J Ophthalmol 2004;88:719–720 Ask the following questions for virtual reality test: 1. Was the test comfortable? If no- How? 2. Was the test too long? 3. How did you find the test? Would you describe it as easy or difficult? If you found it difficult- how? 4. How would you feel if you knew you had to perform this test at every clinic appointment? 5. Do you have any other comments about the test?	Responses from all participants will be collated and summarized at the end of the study, average 1 year.

Sponsor
Queen's University, Belfast

Collaborators
- University of Sussex

Investigators
- Principal Investigator: Ruth E Hogg, PhD, Queen's University, Belfast

General Publications
No publications available

Index

J. N. Weiss, *Clinical Trials in Stargardt Disease Treatment*, https://doi.org/10.1007/978-3-031-58807-5